How to Select the Right Nutritional Supplements for Optimal Health

Mary Esther Miranda Gilbert

ISBN-10: 150084635X
ISBN-13: 978-1500846350

DEDICATION

To Mark and Laura:

May your lives always be vibrant with true health, love, and abundance.

Mary Esther Miranda Gilbert

CONTENTS

PREFACE

How This Book Came About

This book has been the culmination of years of studying and examining ingredients in foods and nutritional supplements, and passing this information on to clients who sought my nutritional consultation services. For their consultation sessions, I would always request that clients bring in their nutritional supplements to my office, where we would review every ingredient listed on those product labels, and they would learn the difference between absorbable, non-absorbable and potentially harmful ingredients. Subsequently, they would discover that most of those boxes or bags full of supplements they brought in were redundant, nutritionally inadequate, nonabsorbable, and/or contained toxic or allergenic ingredients.

Early on, I soon realized that there were not many authoritative, reliable information sources all in one place where people could learn how to choose their supplements effectively. Raising the knowledge and true health awareness on a larger scale in many more millions of people has become more critical, including selecting supplements that truly fill a nutrient void or provide additional nutritional intensity when needed. I wrote this book to turn a three-page educational document I normally provided for my clients on how to select the right supplements into an entire, more in-depth reference guide. This book has been on my To Do list for some time, but a few months ago, one request from an exceptional fitness trainer and associate asking my advice about which nutritional supplements to offer his clientele is what finally sparked the writing of this book. Thank you, Rance of Constant Elevation Fitness!

After completing formal education in nutrition science, human physiology and holistic nutritional healing, and for over thirty-five years of experience as a professional consultant, I developed successful, evidence-based, nutritional health-building protocols for clients who suffered from all manner of ailments. Searching through university, government and other archived scientific literature, I became aware of the vast amount of information about nutritional healing that was not reaching the public. The media, formal nutrition education, and the food and supplement industries left much to be desired for fulfilling the correct nutritional requirements to keep a human being in optimal health and prevent degenerative disease. I remained a watchful consumer advocate over the supplements industry, teaching clients how to pick out the truly useful nutritional supplements from the ones that are a complete waste of time and could actually be harmful.

This book will help you select more absorbable, potent and safe nutrient formulations that can protect you from the degenerative effects of nutrient deficiencies in the food you eat. It will help you protect your health from the disease process if you have been consuming nutrient deficient foods, even if you feel you eat a generally "healthy" diet. Also, knowing the origins of your supplement ingredients is critical to determine just how effective your supplements really are.
Many thousands of people are taking supplements of poor quality. Chances are, those supplements may be doing more harm than good, creating inflammatory

conditions due to the biological incompatibility of synthetic vitamins and the non-absorbable types of minerals used by manufacturers who want to cut production costs. According to the Linus Pauling Institute and other university studies throughout the world, nutrient deficiencies are the major cause of many degenerative diseases millions of people suffer from today, and that includes deficiencies due to poorly formulated supplements.

If you're not eating a completely balanced diet at every meal from food grown or raised in a nutrient and phytonutrient-rich ecosystem such as an organically sustainable, permaculture environment, you are likely missing some essential nutrients that are impairing your optimal health potential. Since the majority of people are not currently eating foods from such an environment, the right nutritional supplements may be warranted. However, selecting the right supplements from the overwhelming numbers of formulations available on the market requires some knowledge of nutrients and the types of those nutrients the human body can utilize. Through the right knowledge, one can easily dismiss the majority of supplements out there and hone in on the ones worth taking.

The main problem in taking supplements is in thinking one's nutrient requirements are being met, when in fact they may not even be absorbing the ones they have chosen, or not being utilized fully if they contain synthetic vitamins or elemental minerals. When the trillions of cells composing the entire human body are being deprived of the right nutrients, be it from poor food choices or poorly absorbed supplements, any one of multiple trillions of interactive, interdependent biochemical processes in those innately intelligent cells may be misdirected or halted.

Chronic deficiency conditions in your biochemistry are where the disease process begins, where symptoms gradually become increasingly debilitating and result in full blown diseases. The only way to reverse this process is to provide the full range of nutrients that originate in nutrient rich soils and that yield nutrient-rich foods that in turn become the ingredients in your supplements, as opposed to a chemical recipe of only a few synthetic and molecularly incomplete ingredients in a biologically inadequate supplement.

Thousands of people are buying supplements that the body cannot utilize or that cause inflammatory responses due to their inability to be absorbed inside human cells, much less utilized properly, yet the products may be purported to have an instant or rapid desired result. There is no such thing as instant health. Through the years as a holistic nutritional consultant, teaching individual clients how to transform their health was effective and successful by redirecting how they chose their supplements and foods, and clients soon learned that there are no shortcuts in the way the body utilizes nutrients.

You get what you pay for in the way of price and nonabsorbability. Mixing synthetic vitamins and finely ground mineral elements and forming them into tablets with toxic binders and excipients does not constitute a healthy supplement, not when natural laws govern how the body's cells require the much more complex molecular structures from whole, energy-active, enzyme-active foods, whose atomically charged atoms are vital in the true life-transferring, life-promoting effect.

If you wish to have truly effective supplements, the ingredients in those formulations must contain whole food, enzyme-active substances in the mix, and one or more combinations of formulations must contain the full range of all known essential nutrients found in whole foods. The ongoing debate over whether supplements are good for you or bad could be quickly settled if this little tidbit would be brought out into the open.

Additionally, isolated nutrients, synthetic or drug-like substances formulated into a so-called magical product that claims to have specific and quick results is usually only temporary at most, and often may produce undesirable side effects. The biochemical pathways the body takes in utilizing chemicals, isolated substances or extracts in many popularized products are more complex than one can imagine and often deceivingly does not and likely cannot produce any claimed and hoped for results. Just because a product appears to work doesn't mean it's something the body can handle for very long. People are getting hurt and being sadly misled, and this book will help put a stop to this madness.

To make matters even more complicated when it comes to deciding whether one should take supplements, you and thousands of people are constantly being inundated with confusing media reports influenced by mega-corporate designs not interested in the least with promoting optimal, true health, which includes non-holistic minded product manufacturers producing supplements without human health interests on their agenda. I am weary of the public constantly receiving the wrong facts about nutritional supplements and nutrition in general, and am dedicated to protecting the reputations of those ethical companies with a sincere desire to improve their customer's health.

By helping you distinguish the difference between poor nutritional supplements and truly efficacious nutritional products that actually promote optimal health, you can also begin to recognize any sensationalized products designed for quick sales that do not offer long term, protective health benefits. You can also begin to distinguish misleading, derogatory reports about supplements or specific nutrients that are broadcasted through the media, such as issuing warning signs of a general nature without actually providing real evidence and adequate details for helping the public make informed decisions. This book is designed to help you recognize how unjustly such bad press is affecting the many ethical, environmentally and sustainability conscious producers of efficacious nutritional supplements who work so hard to earn their deserved customers' trust and continued business.

By keeping people's own nutritional physiology a mystery or making nutritional supplementation a confusing subject, influential corporate designs that impose educational limitations over the masses render millions of individuals much more gullible and vulnerable to the prevalent false dogma and marketing propaganda. By controlling what you see, read and hear, confusing issues with information that is often unscientific, biased, contradictory and misleading, your wellness management becomes overwhelming while information exposed to you is often falsified and incomplete. When you seek information, unless you have had an in-depth education in the sciences, it is difficult to sort the pseudo science from true science.

A perfect design that has been in place for decades, a lifetime of misinformation starts a whole cascading effect in consumer choices that leads one toward the disease process. It is a highly profitable multi-corporate machinery that has become a multi-trillion dollar business, and has made them insanely wealthy and powerful. Health-conscious people have reached the saturation point of tolerance in poor supplements and lack of food quality, and with growing awareness, are turning away from unsatisfying and contradictory information and seeking truth. This book will show you the difference between what are scientifically sound and biologically compatible supplements, and those not worth your time. Your informed choices can help stop irresponsible, inhumane corporations from confusing your health choices and messing with your health any longer.

It is disturbing that media efforts that sensationalize the negative aspects of supplements may ruin the reputations of companies that are responsible, which high ethical standards in their manufacturing of whole food supplements do make a difference in one's health. This book will help you see clearly how sincere companies producing quality nutritional supplements are being lumped in with the poorly formulated supplements of other manufacturing companies through inaccurate and misleading media reporting and are therefore being wrongly represented. Your educated choices are needed to help support the true health advocates producing quality products.

Ironically, opposing industries that lead the public toward the degenerative disease downward spiral that includes tactics that discourage people from integrating nutritional supplements in their wellness management may actually own companies that manufacture nutritional supplements or supply supplement manufacturers with ingredients. This means they both essentially encourage the purchase of nutritional supplements with synthetic and toxic ingredients through the very companies they own or do business with, and then turn around and issue warnings against supplements in the media. In that hypocrisy, they are turning profits on both sides of the coin while building wealth supplying the public with poorly formulated supplements. Go through this entire book and it will become obvious to you that much of the confusing information the average person encounters is unfairly and untruthfully misleading the public away from truly effective and safe supplements because ultimately, it's more profitable to keep the masses uninformed and sick, rather than helping them discover their higher health and vibrancy.

As a result of fear-instilling tactics that affect the entire nutritional supplement industry, generating mass confusion about supplements is putting millions of people's health at risk, even as they think they are protecting their health by purchasing nutritional supplements that may in fact be causing harm. Millions of people are foregoing quality supplements because they are not properly informed, and therefore missing the opportunity to protect or optimize their health with the right selections. It's time to turn this level of underhandedness around to your advantage, for you are the one whose health is at stake.

You may likely be one who is wasting precious, hard earned money on the wrong supplements. When it comes to manufacturers deciding to use non-absorbable, potentially toxic or allergenic ingredients in their supplement formulations and what criteria, if any, improperly informed people use when selecting their supplements, it is of great concern that uncaring corporations may be pushing products on an innocent, trusting public purely for profits.

This book is written with the intent that you acquire the right knowledge to select nutritional supplements that will support your health goals while empowering the true health movement that encourages more nutritional supplements be produced that actually improve health, not put it at risk. Since many supplement manufacturers don't seem to be too concerned with nutrient bioavailability as they are with production costs and using cheap, synthetic ingredients, through your informed purchases, you have the power to help change the nutritional supplements industry and create a greater demand for better supplements.

I created this book because there seem to be no adequate, detailed formal guidelines for health conscious people to follow in selecting supplements, or for knowing which ingredients are actually effective for ensuring health improvement or protection against deficiency diseases and toxicity. This information is scattered, incomplete and often incorrect. In short, this book sets the record straight on which supplements are actually good for you, and which are actually not. This book is intended to educate more people so we as a collective, health advocating, formidable citizen force can influence supplement manufacturers to choose their ingredients and ingredient suppliers more discriminately and socially responsibly.

With the knowledge required to choose the right

supplements, we can, through our purposeful purchases, help create a demand for those ingredient suppliers who focus on sustaining a clean, nutrient rich environment from which supplement ingredients may originate. With the right knowledge empowering you, you can forego choosing incompatible and molecularly incomplete, synthetic versions that create deficiencies and inflammatory conditions in your body, and through your choices, you can discourage the manufacture of supplements designed to promote the profits of those industries not concerned with true cellular nourishment, nor concerned with their customer's optimal health.

This book came about because I want you to experience the peace of mind that comes with knowing you are knowledgeable and able to select the best possible nutritional supplements for your health. I want to ensure that you are qualified to help yourself and others avoid unnecessary products, and to get the most out of those products you do select.

INTRODUCTION

What to Expect From Reading This Book

Use this book as a reliable reference manual to open your eyes to the world of nutritional supplements and the variety of ingredients you will encounter, to learn how ingredients are used by the body, and why many ingredients are commonly included in supplement formulations. This book provides an in-depth look into what you may be putting into your body with your current supplements, and how you are being affected at the micro cell level, where real health is either destroyed or repaired, and rebuilt, maintained and protected. How To Choose The Right Supplements also provides additional reference resources from which to further ensure your knowledge of supplements that may truly serve as an added protective measure in your whole health management protocol.

Getting familiar with its valuable content will save you thousands of dollars in unnecessary nutritional supplement purchases. By not having to be uncertain if you're making the right choices, and being able to slice through the overload of misleading advertising, pseudo-scientific marketing tactics and prevalent, misleading information that may be shrouding over your selections, you will be a more savvy steward and therefore a more effective guardian of your own health.

Those who switch their supplements to those with high potency, nutrient dense and biocorrect ingredients can feel and see the difference in their health, sometimes in one day, and usually within several days as the body begins to utilize essential nutrients at the micro level immediately toward greater functioning. With thorough nutritional supplementation along with a nutrient dense, whole food dietary intake, people typically report improved energy and vitality, and improved overall health.

With follow-up visits to their physician and laboratory tests, a person's values typically improve, such as lowered cholesterol, improved glucose tolerance values, liver enzymes, improved blood pressure, reduced or alleviated pain and inflammation, rapid healing of chronic joint and other structural problems, improved brain and nerve function, alleviated digestive problems, improved skin conditions, and dissolved abnormal growths and tumors. Yes, even cancers have been known to go into remission for indefinite periods, as forbidden as this subject is by the medical industrial complex and the entities that tower over them and oversee all that they do.

I insert the disclaimer here, however, that one should never try to treat their own serious illness or diseased condition without having it diagnosed by a trusted medical practitioner. However, that said, know that I often received clients who felt their physician's courses of treatments were making their health status worse. Clients always signed waivers with the understanding that they were allowing me to design an evidence based nutritional health improvement protocol, and full disclosure to their physician via a form letter was always recommended, though clients often opted out to inform their physicians they were seeking a holistic approach to their health management. It was common that clients had grown disillusioned with the medical system and the attitudes of their physicians when they sought my consult, and that they were very concerned about the rather destructive aftermath of their medical treatments.

When I would show clients the side effects of their prescription drugs, according to the FDA's Medline web site, many of their symptoms they described matched the descriptions of their drugs' side effects. Not being a physician and certainly never intending to pose as one, for interpreting symptoms and drugs are out of my genre of expertise, I would always advise clients to discuss the matter with their own doctors.

This book was not written to discourage you from rejecting Western medicine. However, you must be aware of what runs the medical establishment and be aware of their agendas if you wish to protect your health and your health freedom. To be sure, there are many life-saving medical procedures for which to be thankful, but there are also elements of corruption, medical politics and influences geared toward profit that obstruct many conscientious physicians' ability to practice medicine without putting their patient's health at risk.

However, you are encouraged to discuss with your medical provider the hazardous effects of prescribed drugs, and show him or her this book, for much information about supplements doctors receive concerns synthetic vitamins and elemental minerals, both of which the body cannot readily use. It is no wonder they often do not recommend supplements. I have found through diligent research and investigation into the scientific literature about drug-nutrient side effects that there are few drug-nutrient interactions that may interfere with the effects of a drug, and virtually none appear to be life-threatening, but be sure you and your doctor understand the difference between selecting any supplements containing synthetic or isolated nutrients or extracts and those that are derived from whole food complexes.

Very few whole food supplements are likely to pose a problem with prescribed drugs, since synergistic whole food complexes containing different nutrients are first priority with human cells. Some nutrients reduce or intensify the effects of drugs; some drugs inhibit or amplify certain nutrients, which could affect the performance of a drug.

Therefore, please be sure to discuss these possibilities with your doctor. Do know, however, that the overall health of clients on a complete and correct, full range nutrient supplementation and thorough nutritional dietary protocol always improved, which invariably surprised their doctors, who subsequently took their patient's off their medications or reduced their dosages. The typical physician's remark, according to my clients whose health steadily improved when implementing their new dietary protocol and nutritional supplementation was: "Whatever you're doing, keep doing it.".

This book provides a comprehensive description of the ingredients you will find in a great variety of supplements. You will also learn how the right supplements affect your body's ability to improve the way it handles or eliminates the daily onslaught of thousands of environmental toxic chemicals, and what types of supplements effectively eliminate pathogenic, illness or disease causing micro organisms. You will also find lists of whole food substances with potent detoxification and cell repairing benefits. You will be able to separate the ineffective, incomplete supplements from those that contribute toward your authentic health vibrancy. A full range of naturally derived nutrients are essential for supporting your physical activities, improving mental abilities and the ability to handle stress, and helping to shift the body's biochemistry toward a more optimal state of functioning that has been shown to improve cognition, learning and interpersonal interactions.

By referring to the ingredient descriptions in this book, you can go through your cabinets or cupboards with authoritative confidence and see just how effective your current nutritional supplements are. You will be able to determine if they are incomplete, redundant, non-absorbable, or inadequate for your nutritional needs. If you keep this manual at hand when you go to purchase new supplements, you will come away with only one or just a couple of superior nutritional products that provide the full range of nutrients required by your body to function optimally and improve its inner chemistry. You will find there is no need to keep buying all sorts of partial or potentially harmful, synthetic formulations.

If you keep track of what you spend on nutritional supplements, it is certain that by narrowing your purchase or purchases to the fundamentals outlined here in this manual, you will save time, money and a great deal of ineffectiveness in your choices, and ultimately, save yourself from disappointing results. No matter what your wellness status is currently, there are some very life-enhancing synergistic supplements available that can fill any nutrient voids or deficiencies you might have.

If you are experiencing diminished health, the right choices can make a marked difference in how you feel, particularly if you improve your nutritional food intake. By eliminating toxic chemical ingredients in your food and other toxic consumer product choices, and you begin an exercise program which energy output and nutritional replenishment is in balance with your current state of health, you can continue to see improvement progress toward your greatest possible health and life transformation.

If you are in general good health and feel you are handling life just fine, imagine how much more you could accomplish and how much more abundantly energetic you could feel and youthfully more vibrant you could look if you were to provide your body systems with a higher level of nutrient density and nutritional synergy that inevitably elevates all areas of your life. If your health is "good enough", are you absolutely certain you are not missing essential nutrients that may produce chronic or degenerative symptoms in the near future? Are you beginning to experience signs of the degenerative, deficiency disease process by experiencing any number or types of symptoms? Do you look older than you feel or actually are?

If you are already vibrantly healthy and are energetic and physically fit, this book will serve as a positive reinforcement for your healthy lifestyle and enhance your ability to influence and lead others. How to Choose the Right Supplements also will help ensure that you continue to nourish your body, mind and spirit optimally as you continue throughout your life to remain completely and correctly nourished, perpetuating your biologically youthful state of vibrancy indefinitely, your whole life and well into advanced age.

While true, whole health begins with proper daily whole food nutrition obtained from a nutrient dense, chemical-free environment, the same is true for optimal nutritional supplements which ingredients must also be derived from those same kinds of environments. Devour this manual, cover to cover, and you will become your own best expert when it comes to selecting your nutritional supplements, and be able to protect your health from all of the confusing propaganda out there. When you are well informed about selecting nutritional supplements after utilizing this manual, read my other books and articles about food selections and my unique food system that also ensures you receive a full range of nutrients from expertly combining your food choices.

To your true health,
Esther

1 Why Take Nutritional Supplements

Today's lifestyles are often fast-paced, and with demanding careers, jobs, educational pursuits and other life activities requiring long hours or commutes imposing on one's otherwise personal time, one may feel forced to choose less than optimally nourishing meals on a regular basis and feel there is no time for thoughts about one's nutritional health. Nutritional neglect, abuse or indifference, though may be unintentional, results in an array of inevitable symptoms. Chronic and long term nutrient deficiencies leads to diminished life performance as a person experiences lessened physical work capacity, greater fatigue and lowered mental abilities.

Critical missing dietary nutrients leads to the predictable increase in abnormal physical symptoms such as more frequent illnesses or other body system malfunctions, all of which are signs that the unsuspecting individual has entered the degenerative disease process. Long term nutrient deficiencies so common among populations in developed countries today are the true culprits of the epic proportions of health problems to which millions of individuals have fallen victim. The more people have become disconnected from understanding that the full range of essential nutrients are the absolute foundation of true health, disease prevention and health recovery, the greater the numbers of individuals have suffered unnecessarily.

We can no longer ignore the fact that there is an obesity epidemic that has been and continues to increase at an alarming rate in industrialzied nations. Habitually relying on refined foods, sweets, processed foods, plasticized oils, beverages and fast foods containing toxic ingredients are raising the rate of many types of disease risks to an all time high. The USDA (United States Department of Agriculture) informs us that essential nutrients and protein in the production of at least forty-three whole foods has declined since 1950. Conventional farming practices, through the use of chemical fertilizers, adversely affect the nutrient density and life of soils, as well as diminish habitats and ecosystems in the environment.

People are consuming foods that are grown in soils devoid of essential trace minerals such as chromium, iodine, manganese and selenium, which are required for preventing disease and maintaining optimal health, and are therefore suffering from a variety of nutrient deficiency health conditions. As has been revealed through extensive scientific research and documented literature, nutrients derived from whole foods and quality supplements are required by the body daily and can correct many health conditions (Citizens 2013).

Since conventionally grown foods are deficient in many essential nutrients and can contain genetically modified organisms or sprayed with synthetic, toxic chemicals, we must do all we can to support organic, sustainable farming methods that replenish and recycle rich soils and retain nutrient density in a balanced eco environment. Until more sustainable, permaculture food production methods are implemented, which build and yield soils rich in nutrients that mimic the most fertile areas on Earth, it is wise to take the right nutritional supplements.

The full range of all known essential nutrients should be the basis of any supplement protocol, and should include naturally derived vitamins, absorbable and biocompatible forms of minerals, and a host of phytonutrients and enzymes from whole food ingredients in the plant kingdom. Along with quality protein, fats and nutrient-rich carbohydrate food sources, full range supplementation ensures that any nutrient deficiencies are filled. The human body simply cannot survive, let alone thrive, if there are daily, chronic nutrient deficiencies, and proper supplementation can make all the difference.

In a USDA survey, it was found that over 80% of women and more than 70% of men consumed less than two-thirds the government's Recommended Daily Allowance (RDA) of one or more nutrients daily. Also, it was revealed that although people are eating 20% more vegetables than twenty-five years ago, 25% of those vegetables are prepared in a way as to cause disease, such as those eating artery clogging, cancer causing French fries. There is clear evidence showing that taking a daily multi-nutrient supplement that includes the right forms of vitamins and minerals can reduce the risk of various diseases and therefore one can achieve a higher state of health for a longer period during one's life (Stanford 2000).

Unless you grow your own food sustainably and organically and pay strict attention to building the soil in which it is grown, a variety of fresh fruits, vegetables, nuts, seeds, herbs, whole grains, legumes and other whole food natural nutrient substances such as bee pollen may still be missing vital essential minerals. Relatively few people still do not accomplish an optimal level of nutrition consistently, so nutritional supplementation, along with a well balanced daily food intake, can significantly help reduce nutrient deficiencies that can lead to disease.

Although the U.S. is considered to have the best-fed people in the world, it is only in reference to their calorie intake, and in fact Americans are overfed and undernourished from eating too many nutrient-deficient, empty calorie foods. This is true for adults as well as children. Unfortunately, a great portion of many people's diets consists of cake, cookies, donuts and sugary drinks that degrades any efforts of eating nutritious foods. When it comes to actual life expectancy, Americans are 17th in line while health care costs continue to rise well over $600 billion. Meanwhile, research continues to produce proof that taking mult-vitamin, mineral and other whole food supplements improves health and protects one from disease. Multiple nutrient supplements have cut fetal deaths, low birth weight and pre-term births by 40%, and reduce risk of colon cancer by 75%, according to one nurses' study (Stanford 2000).

Even the FDA has finally conceded that more folic acid is needed by demographical groups such as pregnant women, that folic acid and vitamin B6 reduces heart disease risk by 50%, that higher doses of Vitamin E reduces heart disease rates, and that vitamins C and E reduce infectious diseases among the elderly by 50% compared to those who do not take these supplements. Cancer causes 500,000 American deaths per year, and vitamins A, C and E, along with other essential nutrients, can reduce the risk of acquiring this dreaded disease. Vitamins C and E also have been shown to delay the development of cataracts by at least ten years (Stanford 2000).

With many more thousands of studies with successful health improvement outcomes demonstrating the advantages of taking the right nutritional supplements, it is wise to consider a well-thought out, complete individual nutrient protocol. Things to consider in selecting your nutritional supplements are your gender, age, amount of physical work you do in your job, how often you exercise and the types of exercise you do, your current health status, and dietary habits and preferences. There are disease risks affecting every demographic due to the high levels of toxic chemicals one is exposed to daily from industrial and other sources of pollution, including the toxic effects of agricultural chemicals.

Personal care products containing synthetic ingredients, as well as prescription drugs, nutritional deficiencies and consuming processed foods also raise a person's risk of disease due to their cumulative, nutrient-depleting effect upon the body. Those who have compromised immune systems, are recovering from an illness, surgery or athletic or accidental injury heal more rapidly and thoroughly with nutritional supplements. Nutritional supplementation has a positive effect on mental stress and helps provide nutrients important for the body's ability to produce energy more efficiently.

Due to non-sustainable agriculture, essential-to-life nutrients, particularly a full range of minerals, are chronically missing from farmland soils, resulting in nutrient-deficient food crops. With such depletion of nutrients, fresh foods have been nutritionally inadequate for satisfying the nutritional requirements of human beings and animals for several decades. Poorly managed soils contribute to poorly retained soil moisture, release green house gases and lose nutrients during rains and irrigation. With a great amount of chemical fertilizers, herbicides and pesticides being washed away that end up polluting waterways and water tables, it can be argued that nutritional supplementation with higher nutrient potencies than the government's Recommended Daily Allowance (RDAs) and those supplements with detoxifying value are much needed for protecting you against the diseases caused by the daily onslaught of toxic chemical pollutants.

2 Why Nutritional Supplements are Vital For You to Thrive

The Many Causes of the Current Disease Epidemic

Nutrient density has become more important than ever before if we humans hope to reverse the health effects of the thousands of toxic chemicals we are exposed to daily, for it is the potent nutrients and phytonutrients found in nature's whole foods that are able to detoxify and protect the body from the many common diseases and health disorders people suffer with today. There has been a steady increase in human diseases that correlates with the increased amounts of synthetic chemicals we are exposed to daily. Therefore, concentrated nutrients in their correct biological forms are warranted against the overwhelming onslaught of chemical toxicity that conventional farming and food processing just cannot provide.

Common degenerative diseases in the present day are also the result of years of chronic nutrient deficiencies and nutritional abuse. More scientific studies continue to reveal that many common diseases people suffer from are the result of nutrient-depleted processed foods and their synthetic ingredients. More studies are also showing that toxic chemicals that have adverse affects on health are present in the soil, water and air as the result of industrial pollution. Conventionally grown food crops that are constantly sprayed with chemical pesticides, and many foods that are transgenically altered with genetically modified organisms (GMOs) in an attempt to make crops insect resistant are now linked to genetic defects, cancer, and brain and nervous system disorders.

To complicate matters, poor health is often the result of the abundant misinformation and lack of informing the public about the true nature of how the human body works and the types and forms of nutrients it needs to prevent the many common diseased health conditions in the first place. Corporate control of the information the public receives through the media, education, and many other perspectives is geared toward selling people on false dogma about their health that leads them down the path of disease for the sake of profit.

Complete and correct nutrition is vital at the micro cell level, where true health occurs. Therefore, a strong foundational knowledge of one's own nutritional physiology has become a critical necessity in order to see through the veil of false information and manipulative ploys one constantly encounters, often unbeknownst to the unwary, trusting or innocent individual. The following section demonstrates what you are actually up against when trying to make sound decisions about your health, of which you may not even aware, where even selecting your nutritional supplements becomes a challenge.

Protecting Your DNA Against GMOs

Unlike many European countries that have either banned GMO agricultural production entirely or instituted mandatory labeling laws, GMO labeling is currently not required of product manufacturers and agricultural crops in the U.S., although grass roots movements are continually making progress in enacting change. More food and supplement companies are voluntarily labeling their products with "Non-GMO" claims. In Hawaii, GMO crops have recently been banned at this point in time, after California and Washington States have lost ballot initiatives for mandatory labeling of GMO foods by very close margins, and other countries have also bannedGMOs.

Although national polls indicate that over 90% of Americans favor mandatory GMO labeling laws, and want to know what they are putting into their bodies and how it is affecting their ability to prevent disease, millions of dollars spent by corporations with vested interests on counter measures confusing the public and influencing their votes against mandatory labeling has impeded progress. Unlike other countries, the U.S. lags seriously behind when it comes to protecting the health of its citizens, and the severe complacency in its population has been a challenge in mobilizing enough people to effect more rapid change.

In spite of limited funding compared to the massive wealth of mega corporations behind the production of toxic pesticides and unregulated biotechnology experimenting with GMOs in the food supply and evading environmental responsibilities, grass roots movement efforts and their distribution of educational materials through information networks indicate it is only a matter of time before GMO mandatory labeling laws are implemented throughout the U.S., or banned from agricultural production altogether.

It is a dire matter of how quickly the citizens of any country can stand up to the financial power of those entities that are killing millions of people and wreaking havoc on critical ecosystems that affect everyone on a global scale. Laboratory studies showing the link between cancer and other possible diseases from consuming GMO foods have largely been kept from the public eye. Below is a list of foods that may appear in nutritional supplements in whole food form or as extracts or partitioned portions of whole foods that may contain GMOs.

List of GMO Ingredients and Their Derivatives Crops to Avoid Unless They Are Organically Grown

- Soy
- Alfalfa
- Corn (includes corn sweeteners)
- Zucchini
- Sugar beets (usually listed on labels as "sugar")
- Tomatoes
- Dairy (animals fed GMO feeds)
- Canola oil
- Salmon (may affect wild non-GMO salmon once released into the environment)

- Potatoes

Deadly Synthetics

Other human diseases have been linked to the outgassing from plastic bottles of Bisphenol-A (BPA) and bisphenol-S (BPS). These substances leach these toxins into the water in those containers, particularly if left exposed to high temperatures outdoors in the sun or in a car during hot weather months, and are also released into canned foods that are lined with these volatile chemicals. The massive amounts and accumulation of bisphenols A and S from plastic bottles and many other pollutants that have been dumped into the ocean can be found in the tissues of sea life along the entire food chain, which means humans are consuming these toxic substances too. Ocean currents known as gyres have resulted in land mass size accumulations of plastic debris in the Pacific ocean, and motions of the gyres prevent the trash from escaping. These masses covering hundreds of square miles have are known as The Great Pacific Garbage Patch, The Eastern Pacific Garbage Patch, or the Pacific Trash Vortex. Those toxic polymers have disrupted other entire ecosystems as well as they have found their way to other water sources.

Other synthetic toxic chemicals contained in most personal care and household products are absorbed into the skin and lungs and are retained in fatty tissues, including the brain. These toxic affronts to the human body are cumulative from each generation to the next, with each generation acquiring an ever increasing body burden of chemicals disrupting hormone or endocrine gland functioning, causing nervous system and brain/memory/learning disorders, cancer, birth defects and other diseases plaguing entire societies today.

Never before in the history of humankind has it been more critical to our species' survival that we take immediate action toward reversing the damage we have caused to our very genetic code. To further degrade the diminishing human genome or the genetic code of our species before it can no longer perpetuate itself in optimal functioning and health, people must reexamine what they are putting into their bodies and the consequences of the products they use every day. Simply by choosing whole, nutrient dense and phytonutrient-rich foods grown organically and with sustainability as first priority, and by choosing products that do not contain ingredients that harm you will continue to encourage the shift in entire industries toward healthier humans and a cleaner world.

You, the consumer, are the one who leads those industries to behave responsibly or irresponsibly, for they all want your consumer dollars, will sell you anything you're willing to buy, and care not for the long term consequences. If you want instant gratification as they do, that is all that matters to them, even if it eventually kills you. Whether we have realized this or not, we, that is, the entire world population, can no longer continue to affect the Earth's natural resources on which we all depend for our sustenance, including breathing air, drinking water, and eating food that does not cause disease. We must see the connection between our health and the health of the planet, or we vanish as a species, along with the diversity of life that has been here around us for thousands of years.

Because of our innocence, ignorance or indifference, stubborn reliance on fossil fuels with our sweeping-under-the-rug attitude, we have caused a tragic imbalance in entire ecosystems throughout the world as a result. We now must face the increasing violence of the natural forces of nature, which includes more severe weather, global warming from increasingly greater amounts of desertification that has resulted in greater flooding and increasing amounts of melting polar ice caps. Continuing our irresponsible, non-sustainable monoculture farming methods, burying plastic containers that literally creates mountains of non-biodegradable trash, and ocean dumping, fracking, thoughtless deforestation of rainforests and other forests and creating more non-revivable deserts, industrial pollution and toxic food choices adds up to one thing. We are destroying ourselves rapidly and destroying the natural world that we need in order to not only stay alive, but thrive in full cooperation with its natural laws.

More Sustainability in Food Production Needed - But Without Exploitation

Our choices have contributed to our epidemic of diseases in our so-called well-fed nations. We use consumer products or consume foods that are produced by exploited workers and indebted farmers. Our choices, be they innocent or indifferent, have contributed to the making of dependent, starving nations that were previously self-sufficient. Furthermore, until more of us realize how crucial it is to economically and locally support time-proven organic sustainable farming and the holistic management and raising of livestock, the superior nutrient value of our food supply and abundant crop yields cannot take back their rightful places on the planet. Our choices must support sustainable methods to produce enough abundance for providing all of our nutrient needs without destroying the interdependent, life diversity we humans have historically benefited from for thousands of years.

With our disruption of the delicate chain of life, we have caused entire ecosystems to cascade into environmental devastation over and over again throughout history. In our unrelenting consumption, we have turned forests into deserts, health into disease. Each time humans have done this, the Earth's ability to recuperate has been diminished, just as a person whose body is sick with diminishing resources loses the ability to recover from degeneration and illness. The Earth is overwhelmed with toxic wastes and barren lands and is having trouble recovering, and its powerful backlash as it tries to right itself is having increasingly violent consequences on our lives and that of all living things.

As a species, if we do not focus on a whole ecology, human beings lack of foresight and vision when it comes to food production will continue to turn lush and water-abundant green lands into more deserts. A sustainable and thriving environmental approach to food production that includes preventing soil erosion and maintaining nutrient density means higher quality ingredients in your nutritional supplements. Without attention to protecting soil fertility by farmers, and without consumers making the necessary food and supplement choices to encourage such sustainable, replenishment practices, quality ingredients derived from nutrient dense, organic food sources is likely to diminish.

Grass roots organizations' and holistic minded professionals' efforts to influence an economic and health-conscious shift in consumer purchases to nutrient-rich nutritional supplements produced by ethical companies is constantly intercepted by less ethical, indifferent corporations single-mindedly selling billions of synthetic supplements without regard to optimal health. These two versions of nutritional supplement production is not apparent to the innocent consumer seeking to improve his or her health with supplementation.

Mass Confusion About Supplements

Profit corporate agendas generate self-serving, far reaching propaganda in every avenue of distribution, including ensuring no medical professional training includes knowledge about nutrients and their essential health-protective, disease-preventing benefits. There is very little appropriate educating of consumers through the media about essential nutrients, and is effectively negating the proper decisions consumers need to make when choosing their supplements. There are no established guidelines for consumers as to which types of supplement ingredients are more effective, and there is an overwhelming amount of contradicting information because true scientific facts are minimized, distorted, or completely ignored in the name of competitive consumer sales.

Various industries have tapped into the billion dollar consumer market of nutritional supplements, including the pharmaceutical industry. With no true interest in human vibrancy and true health, these industries leave the consumer vulnerable to purchasing supplements containing toxic ingredients derived from various industries whose products are linked to disease-causing chemicals and genetically modified organisms (GMOs). Ironically, millions of innocent consumers purchase a wide array of nutritional products that may only contain very few or inadequate amounts of essential nutrients the body may not be able to absorb, and are still not satisfying their body's desperate need for effective nutrients.

Why throw money away, literally, down the toilet by taking poorly formulated supplements. Elemental mineral supplements, for instance, end up bogging down sewage waste facilities as they must constantly remove often fully intact, undigested calcium tablets. Back in the seventies, I used to take oyster shell calcium tablets, until one enlightening day after an x-ray taken by my chiropractor showed the tablet, fully intact, on its way out of my digestive tract.

Costly advertising dollars are encouraging millions of people to manage their nutritional health with inadequate, incomplete nutritional advice and heavily leading people toward relinquishing and deferring any health decisions to drug industry-influenced professionals who mistrust the authentic nutrient substances needed for supporting life and helping it thrive. Choosing the right supplements and typically feeling and seeing the improved health results only confirms the vast amounts of scientific data that helps disprove any misinformed objections by those who have not been properly informed or those who have any agendas that reward them for opposing the real facts about supplements. Only educating consumers as to which supplement ingredients actually improve health and which do not can influence the necessary market shift toward the truly health-improving supplements while promoting better product label ingredient disclosure.

Investing in whole food, bio-compatible nutritional supplements, rather than non-absorbable, incomplete formulations containing potentially toxic ingredients actually can mean the difference between a successful health management protocol, and one that does not protect against nutrient-deficiencies, leaving one susceptible to many physical ailments and preventable diseases. A correctly informed health-conscious consumer is the solution for ultimately improving the quality and efficaciousness of more nutritional supplements, for informed consumers demand and purchase nutritionally superior products, forcing less than optimal supplement producers to improve their ingredients to meet consumer demands if they wish to stay in business.

Sustainability in Food Production Equals Better Supplements

Purchasing supplements with synthetic ingredients not only spells trouble for your body's trillions of cells, it means less business for the organic, sustainable food production industry that actually improves rather than destroys vital environments that yield nutrient dense food materials used in truly nourishing supplements. Less organic sustainable food production means less nutrient-rich whole foods and supplements for you to use to protect yourself against the many dietary and environmental causes of disease. With deforestation having a devastating effect on essential ecosystems that would otherwise help ensure food abundance on the planet, and the disconnectedness and unawareness of the vital importance of nature in which many people live their lives, it is wise for consumers to make choices that help reverse this increasingly threatening and dire predicament in which we human beings have caused for ourselves.

Consumer purchases are certainly what drives markets, and choosing products with better ingredients surely helps ensure greater health and protection against deficiency diseases. Our choices can make or break the organic, sustainable agriculture industry. If we do not support them, our health and health freedom choices are at stake. Therefore, no matter what, the more we consumers support the safe food production and protection of local and worldwide, nested ecosystems that produce higher nutrient-dense crops from which supplements are made, the more you can ensure not succumbing to a deficiency disease.

If we support organic farms which farmers manage the land sustainably, large operations and small alike, we have a greater chance of gaining the critical awareness of the importance of cooperating with nature, rather than arrogantly trying to control and conquer it. If one chooses synthetic and toxic supplements, that is one less person contributing toward maintaining the vital planetary ecosystems that determine the quality of the air we breathe, how clean our water is, and how nutrient-rich an environment is where food is grown or raised.

Insisting on choosing poorly absorbed or non-absorbable supplements to save money may only increase your medical bills and consequently cause unnecessary psychological trauma for all involved. With so many people choosing inadequate supplements, it's no wonder supplements have sometimes gotten a bad rap. Those whose monetary or self-interests are served by criticizing supplements are the first to renounce the validity of supplementation, even as there is a great amount of scientific evidence that continues to increase that reveals proper nutritional supplementation's impressive effectiveness. The notion of synthetic nutrients is an oxymoron, so buying synthetic supplements because you want to be health conscious doesn't make any sense, especially if you buy organic foods. Selecting useless supplements along with being proud of buying organic foods is inconsistent and self-contradictory.

Millions of people are making daily nutritional choices that have an immediate and long term effect on their health, and because of those choices, made either purposely or innocently, they are suffering the health consequences. Choosing the right supplements means not only accelerating any healing process or helping to maintain health vibrancy, it also means your choices help support interdependent ecosystems that maintain a diversity and abundance of life in environments where thriving habitats play an essential role in the nutritional health-building and health-protecting value of your food. The more consistent a consumer you are in making both health-conscious and environmentally conscious product choices, the more you ensure your own thriving and that of billions of species that can synergistically ensure an abundance of Earth's food and renewable resources indefinitely.

By supporting the organic agriculture and supplement manufacturing industries that produce whole food, nutrient dense and bio-available nutrients, you play an essential role in planetary health and assures your continued thriving. Sustainable agricultural methods keep green house gases carbon, nitrogen and methane from being released into the atmosphere, and recapture them back into the soils where they belong where they are utilized properly by beneficial organisms in the soil and plants. Such soil and plant activity supports rich, living soils that hold pure water and high amounts of nutrients, while forming and preserving healthy water sources that support a diversity of life living interdependently and in synergy. This results in superior nutritional supplements being derived from foods found to be higher in nutrients and from healthier, humanely raised animals grazing on nutrient-rich pastures and fed nutrient-rich feeds.

Among other toxic food and product choices, when you select synthetic supplements, you are having a much greater impact on your world than you might think, having a hand in fueling a negative cascading effect that increases your impact on the world's ecology already in danger of destroying all life on the planet in just a couple of generations. If your supplements contain chemical preservatives and additives better left to clean your car or polish your furniture with, or if they contain genetically modified organisms that would never occur in nature and are known to confuse your cells' DNA genetic code sequencing, it would be wise to simply dispose of them. Unless you support the organic sustainable food production industry, your otherwise toxic choices adversely impact your health and diminish the critical, synergistic symbiosis of all living things, and the less access you have to powerful healing, restorative, regenerative nature's medicines that safely and effectively protect your health as they have done for human beings for thousands of years.

Through encouraging and supporting the synthetic chemical production mindset with what you eat, put on your body, inhale or drink, you diminish your health and environment upon which you depend. By buying nutritional supplements containing toxic ingredients, current conventional agriculture is encouraged to continue polluting the environment, destroying biodiversity and producing chemically-laden foods that cause hormonal disruptions leading to obesity and associated disease risks such as heart disease, hypertension and diabetes. Toxic food production is also linked to birth defects, brain and nervous system disorders and other conditions that can be prevented or alleviated with a daily diet free of toxic chemicals and rich in the full range and adequate potencies of essential nutrients and detoxifying, DNA-correcting phytonutrients.

By making informed choices in your food and nutritional supplement selections, you can help prevent toxic chemical manufacturers from succeeding with ever increasing their profit interest ties with other disease producing industries that control the distribution of toxic substances and continue to be the culprits that are causing a sick, dumbed down populace. Now is not the time, and in fact it has never been the right time, to purchase cheap, toxic nutritional supplements that do not improve your health and in fact harm you and your environment.

3 Choosing The Right Ingredients For The Right Reasons

Nutritional supplement ingredients vary in their biological compatibility with human cells, so care must be taken to choose those that can actually be utilized, rather than create circulatory inflammatory conditions throughout the body due to non-absorbability.

Nutritional multi-nutrient supplements work more intricately and effectively when they are free of synthetic versions of vitamins and non-absorbable elemental minerals, and do not contain toxic or potentially allergenic ingredients. By contrast, their naturally derived vitamin and plant-derived mineral counterparts are found in whole foods grown organically or in ecologically balanced, bio-diverse environments that maintain fertile, nutrient-rich soils. Such nutrients, when formulated into well-designed nutritional supplements, are biocompatible and non-toxic, and easily recognized by the innately discriminating microscopic cell membranes when the nutrients arrive for cell entry and then allowed to proceed with the trillions of biochemical processes that occur within those cells.

The cell membrane is the innately intelligent, protective gateway into the powerful manufacturing facilities within each cell that directs how accurately your cells replicate, divide, and perpetuate your existence, and where your genetic code within the DNA double helix is housed protectively. Within each cell are the powerful factories where the quality of cell functioning depends on the quality of nutrients you take in, and determines their level of ability to repair damaged cells and correct any defects to your genetic code. Cells are the units of life that compose the entire body's organs, fluids and structures, and the brain and nervous system. Cell components create new essential proteins, including thousands of protein structures, including regulating and reproductive hormones and enzyme catalysts responsible for stimulating the body's multiple trillions of daily biochemical processes that keep you alive.

Bio-compatible nutrients derived from whole food sources are easily utilized for the repair, regeneration and protection of all interactive, mutually monitoring systems that make up the entire human body. The synthetic, chemical versions of many nutrients are specifically designed with limited specifications within the dynamic rules of chemistry and are inert, relatively simplistic structures the body can interpret as inadequate and likely to reject. Synthetic or laboratory concocted "nutrients" are poor representations of the more complex molecular and atomic arrangements of atoms in their naturally derived, whole food forms, provided the nutrients have not been altered or destroyed during processing. Therefore, the natural laws of nutrient synergy apply to whole food derived supplements, which ingredient sources are carefully harvested and processed to preserve nutrients and enzymes to maintain optimal potency and absorbability.

When selecting an ideal supplement, its effectiveness can be immediately determined upon examining the ingredients on the product label, and the cost versus benefits must be weighed regarding its monetary cost compared to its health-enhancing, health-protective value. The question that you must ask yourself in selecting nutritional supplements is: as a wise health investment, how well can this addition to my daily nutrient intake fulfill any possible nutrient deficiencies and help protect against environmental, chemical toxicity? To prevent or at least minimize future health problems, including a well-chosen nutritional supplement protocol in your health management plan is one of the most fundamental choices you make that can also avert monumental medical costs, and psychological and emotional trauma associated with disease. The disastrous health effects of long-term nutrient deficiencies and the affect on the quality of your life and that of those close to you can be simply avoided through supplementing a whole foods diet and a full range of daily nutrient replenishment through nontoxic, naturally absorbable supplements.

An ideal nutritional supplement program should only include the foundational essential vitamins and minerals in their most absorbable, bio-available form, and also contain whole food, phytonutrient-rich, enzyme-active ingredients. Therefore, the first item on your nutritional supplement list should be a multi-nutrient supplement product that includes the full range of known essential vitamins, a full complement of essential, absorbable minerals, plus active, digestive enzymes and essential fatty acids--all in a base of powders from whole fruits, leafy greens and/or dark green, yellow and red vegetables. An even more complete supplement may contain other whole food components such as herbs or other nutraceuticals or botanicals, amino acids, plant sterols, bee products, blue-green algae, or other organically produced, nutrient dense, whole food items. With such a full range nutrient-dense supplement, it would hardly be necessary to add much more in the way of supplementation.

However, let us first focus on the fundamental essential vitamins and minerals needed for supporting all cellular processes within your trillions of cells in your entire body. Then we can focus on the various possible combinations of whole food ingredients that can improve on your basic vitamin/mineral formulation in many purposeful ways. It is important to know, however, that there are no shortcuts when it comes to your health. With countless nutrient devoid nutritional supplements on the market, a little knowledge about how the body utilizes nutrients and one glance at a product's ingredient list should be all you need to determine if a supplement is worth taking.

To take your choice in supplements another step further, you can call the toll free number on the product label or visit their website and ask them some direct questions about where they source their ingredients from, and whether or not the product contains GMOs. You can also choose your supplements based on their carbon footprint: were the ingredients locally grown or were they transported long distances using great amounts of fossil fuels; were pesticides, herbicides or synthetic fertilizers used on the crops; were the ingredients organically grown and were fair trade practices maintained.

The more a company is willing to disclose to the public, the more trustworthy they become. The more a consumer asks such questions, the more concerned a company becomes about their ethics and manufacturing practices. The more health-conscious people find their voice in expressing what they want and do not want in their supplements, the more the industry will respond competitively to capture your business while perhaps finding their conscience and feeling good about it. Those companies that pass your rigorous analysis can be proud that they are servicing the true health needs of their fellow human beings, are a good example for the supplements industry, and have won your approval and loyalty.

Building and maintaining optimal health means adhering to the universal laws of nature under which the human body is designed. The only way to build true, vibrant health and protect yourself from the disease process is to apply the following tenets on a daily or weekly basis.

- Consume whole, unprocessed foods grown without toxic chemicals, and in nutrient-rich soils irrigated with non-polluted water.
- Nourish the body daily and thoroughly in a timely manner with a balance of the energy nutrients: lean protein, unprocessed whole food fats and whole food carbohydrates, and maintain proper hydration by drinking plenty of purified water.
- Protect the body with an abundance of plant-derived foods containing a wide range of phytonutrients that

strengthen immunity, help cells produce energy, detoxify and eliminate toxic chemicals, repair damaged genetic material in the DNA and help maintain proper electrolyte balance and hydration.

- Include a holistic balance of regular exercise that strengthens muscles, builds strength and cardiovascular endurance, maintains flexibility, and develops whole body coordinated movements such as sports, or physical arts such as dance or martial arts, or other physical activities.
- Balance meaningful work, be a lifelong learner, and live a vibrantly healthy, satisfying life of your own design. Develop keen interests or hobbies, participate in meaningful community and social activities, discover enjoyable things to do and feed your life passions.
- Spend time in nature and set aside time to think, sort things out, put things into perspective, and attend to your spiritual needs.
- Find ways to serve or protect fellow Earth inhabitants; remain conscious of the impact you make on others and in the world; foster satisfying relationships.

A person is best able to accomplish the above tenets of optimal health through raising the energetic efficiency of every single cell in the entire body. What healers have known throughout time and the scientific field of biophysics confirms is that the human body is enveloped in its own bioenergy field, and vibrates at various energy frequencies, the rate at which is determined by one's current state of health. A person who manages their health according to and in cooperation with the universal laws of nature by applying the above tenets vibrates and emits energy at a higher frequency, which correlates with a higher level of physical, mental, emotional and psychological health. The lower one's state of health, the lower the frequency at which one vibrates and emits energy (Bischof 2005).

The body is composed of 65-90% water, depending on the type of cell and the person's age and physical condition. The average water weight of a healthy male is around 42 kilograms, and is composed of 21% protein and 7% bone minerals. The average healthy adult has approximately 12 kg of fat and 12 kg of body protein, which includes not only muscle tissue, but also the proteins that compose the blood, organs, tissues, and countless biochemicals needed for trillions of cellular processes (Rowett n.d.). These numbers vary according to gender, age, state of health and amount and incidence of physical fitness activities.

The human body is also composed of oxygen, carbon, hydrogen, nitrogen, the major minerals calcium, phosphorus, sodium, potassium, sulfur, and the trace minerals magnesium, iron, copper, chlorine and zinc. The body's blood sugar in the form of glucose is converted to its complex carbohydrate, glycogen, as temporary energy reserves stored in muscle cells, to be converted back to glucose again and released into the bloodstream as needed. The utilization of these essential nutrients vary according to individual nutritional habits with food and nutrient choices and type of physical activity.

Considering that we are composed of the above substances and that they are found throughout nature in all living things, and that they are what keeps us optimally alive and functioning besides the air we breathe and the water we drink, it is obvious that we should regularly replenish those things to keep all systems functioning optimally. Nutrients are lost through elimination, perspiration, respiration, and through the endless metabolic processes the body performs every microsecond of our lives that keep us moving, thinking and doing, and such essential nutrients must be replenished on a daily basis and distributed throughout the day through balanced meals and supplements.

With nutrient devoid soils in which the majority of food is currently grown, particularly major and trace minerals, nutrient deficiency diseases in many populations are very common. A bio-correct nutritional supplement containing absorbable forms of essential minerals is therefore warranted. Since essential trace minerals are especially difficult to obtain through the average diet, a nutritionally superior multi-nutrient supplement should also contain them. The chart below lists the essential elements the human body is composed of in descending order.

Body Composition by Elements

Element	Percent By Mass (The total molecular mass of a molecule.)
Oxygen	65
Carbon	18
Hydrogen	10
Nitrogen	3
Calcium	1.5
Phosphorus	1.2
Potassium	0.2
Sulfur	0.2

Chlorine	0.2
Sodium	0.1
Magnesium	.05
Iron, Cobalt, Copper	<0.05 each
Zinc, Iodine	<0.05 each
Selenium, Fluorine	<0.01 each
(Helmenstine 2013)	

The first three elements, oxygen, carbon and hydrogen, combine to form many variations of sugars that participate in trillions of bodily processes, and nitrogen is essential for forming countless protein molecules for repair, growth and perpetuation of energy and cellular life cycles. As minute as the needs of the body are for the above minerals, deficiency disease would soon set in if they were missing in the daily diet. A highly nutrient intensive, biocompatible nutritional supplement helps ensure you leave no stone unturned when it comes to your health and well being, and the prevention of nutritional deficiency diseases.

4 Ingredients in a Well-Chosen, Multi-Nutrient Supplement or Group of Supplements

This section describes each nutrient's functional role in the body, some or most of which may or may not be included in a single multi-nutrient formulation. It is very important to know, however, that since nutrients found in nature are synergistic, and to prevent nutritional imbalances that may produce undesirable effects, it is wise to never take any one nutrient in isolation. Multi-nutrient formulas are always best for greater absorption and utilization.

Vitamins

The best source of vitamins come from naturally-occurring whole foods grown in nutrient-rich environments with plenty of sunlight for vitamin synthesis. The next best source of vitamins come from those same nutrient dense foods. Vitamin supplements with the NOS designation on product labels, or Naturally Occurring Standard, indicate that naturally-occurring nutrient sources from whole foods are somewhat lower in potency than synthetic supplements. However, whole food supplements are much more easily assimilated and 100% usable, and do not result in aggravating body systems or have toxic side effects as do those supplements containing synthetic vitamins (Clement, 2006).

Vitamins are organic micronutrients found in whole foods that are vital for all biochemical processes the human body must perform daily, and essential for preventing disease and perpetuating optimal health. Although vitamins are not energy-providing nutrients like proteins, fats or carbohydrates are, they act in synergy with enzymes, coenzymes, antioxidants and mineral cofactors to complete trillions of specialized, essential functions.

Because vitamins are not manufactured by the human body, they are called essential, and must be derived from whole foods where all vitamin cofactors and vitamin complexes are intact in order to perform their vital functions correctly. As discussed in the Synthetic Version of Vitamins in Chapter 6, there is a vital difference between the whole vitamin compounds found in whole foods versus a synthetic version of a vitamin where only part of the vitamin complex is extracted from its whole food version. Such incomplete molecular structures result in the body searching for a way to complete the fragmented molecule, or attempts to disassemble and eliminate it.

If a part of a food's vitamin complex is isolated and integrated into its synthetic version, the body treats it very differently, much as it would a drug. Perceiving it as a threat and invasion, setting off defense systems and creating more nutrient deficiencies forces the body to use its own resources to complete the missing factors, only to create a net result of nutrient shortages. Such chronic deficiencies can affect the immune system, where it can be compromised enough to result in illness or disease. Synthetic versions of vitamin complexes that occur naturally in fresh foods can no longer be considered a vitamin by its true definition (Clement, 2006).

Vitamins are co-enzymes essential to life, and are called "essential" because the body cannot manufacture them on its own. Vitamins as co-enzymes are involved in metabolism or the rate at which cells convert food to energy. Vitamins are required for forming new cells and to perform all biological processes, including digestion. Vitamins are needed for building an optimally functioning immune and hormonal system, performing muscular work, and maintaining the brain and nervous system. Vitamin C and the B complex vitamins are water-soluble, which means the body cannot store them, so they need to be consumed daily. Fat soluble vitamins are able to be stored in fatty tissue and the liver for longer periods. Examples of fat soluble vitamins are: A, D, and E.

Water Soluble Vitamins

Vitamin C - Acts as an antioxidant, protecting cells from free radical damage. Needed to make collagen to repair injuries, improves the absorption of calcium and iron, plays a major role in immune system functioning.

The B Complex Vitamins:

1. **Thiamine (B1)** - Plays a role in the energy cycle, helps coordinate muscle and nerve activity, supports proper heart functioning, improves circulatory system.
2. **Riboflavin (B2)** - Protects cells from oxidation damage, supports cell energy production, helps convert carbohydrates to glucose, helps convert Vitamin B6 and Folate into usable forms, essential for body growth and red cell production.
3. **Niacin (B3)** - Consists of niacinamide and nicotinic acid. Involved in digestion, converting food to energy, helps form healthy skin, essential for nervous system functioning.
4. **Folate** (Also known as Folacin or Folic Acid) - Prevents anemia, helps produce and maintain new red blood cells, including accurate and rapid cell division, needed to make DNA and RNA, prevents damage to DNA that may lead to cancer, maintains normal homocysteine levels to prevent heart attacks.
5. **Pyridoxine (Vitamin B6)** - Helps produce antibodies against foreign pathogens, normal nerve function, hemoglobin-carrying oxygen, in red blood cells, helps prevent anemia, needed to break down proteins, helps maintain normal blood sugar (glucose) levels.

6. **Cyanocobolamin (Vitamin B12)** - Required for metabolic processes, formation of red blood cells, maintaining nervous system.
7. **Biotin** - Essential for growth, helps break down foods for energy, assisting in metabolism, helps regulate cholesterol, plays a role in the production of hormones.
8. **Pantothenic Acid** - Works closely with biotin in digestion and absorption and energy production, helps regulate cholesterol, helps produce hormones.
9. **Choline** - Used in the synthesis of phospholipids, which are essential for all cell membranes and formation of all messenger molecules, involved in neurotransmission for muscles and memory, prevents fat accumulation in the liver and high cholesterol.

Fat Soluble Vitamins

To ensure optimal absorbability and minimize toxicity, always follow the manufacturer's dosage suggestions on the label when it comes to fat soluble vitamin intakes, and select products with whole food-derived sources, rather than their synthetic versions.

Vitamin A - A group of compounds essential for vision, bone growth, reproduction, cell division and differentiation, helps regulate the immune system and fight off infections, helps destroy viruses, bacteria, promotes healthy eyes, lungs, kidneys, intestines.

Vitamin D - Helps maintain strong bones, formed in the body when skin is exposed to sunlight as Vitamin

D3 or cholecalciferol, helps calcium absorption, prevents osteoporosis, rickets, osteomalacia, involved in nerve to muscle transmission for muscular movement, helps immune system destroy invading viruses, bacteria and other illness-causing micro-organisms.

Vitamin E - Antioxidant, protects cells from free radical damage from pollution and chemicals, helps immune system destroy viruses and bacteria, prevents blood clotting in arteries, helps increase blood vessel diameter, essential for cell-to-cell communication.

Vitamin K - Plays a major role in blood clotting preventing excess bleeding and in developing strong bones, strengthens blood vessels and helps maintain their pliability to prevent bruising and excessive swelling when injured. Prevents the breakdown of tissues indicated by sagging skin.

Minerals

Minerals are cofactors and important constituents in metabolism as essential catalysts that activate enzymes needed for every biochemical and bodily process. In order for the body to effectively utilize and absorb minerals properly, they must be in plant derived form, or included in a molecule that is allowed to pass into the cell membrane. Minerals are primarily stored in the bone, teeth and muscle tissue and have a key role in maintaining body fluid osmotic pressure, which affects water regulation, solutes, acid-base or acid-alkaline equilibrium and blood pressure in the body. Minerals are part of the structure of soft tissues, are vital in nerve impulse transmissions and muscle contractions, including the heart.

Minerals are essential components of vitamins, enzymes and hormones. Minerals are involved in maintaining the pH or acid-alkaline equilibrium in the body. Examples of major minerals predominantly needed in the body are: boron, calcium, chloride, magnesium, phosphorus, potassium, sodium and sulfur. Examples of trace minerals needed in minute amounts are: chromium, copper, iodine, iron, manganese, selenium, and zinc. The major essential to life minerals, also called macro minerals, are needed in larger amounts than the essential trace minerals, known as micro minerals. The form of minerals in any multi-nutrient formulation is what determines its absorbability and usefulness.

Absorbable forms of minerals include:

- A chelated mineral, where the mineral is molecularly bound to an amino acid
- A mineral citrate, where a mineral is bound to vitamin C
- A mineral gluconate, which binds a mineral to a salt, ester or anionic form of gluconic acid. Gluconic acid is a mild organic acid derived from glucose, which is a basic component of whole food carbohydrates.

Poorly absorbed or non-absorbable minerals include:

- Elemental minerals. If the label's ingredients on a product list only the mineral itself and not as a chelate, citrate or gluconate, chances are it will pass through the entire gastrointestinal digestive tract and be eliminated out of the colon. This is especially true for oyster shell calcium tablets. As mentioned earlier, sewage treatment plants filter out thousands of undissolved elemental mineral tablets that have passed through the entire intestinal tract unabsorbed.

- Carbonated minerals such as calcium carbonate or dolomite actually reduce the amount of the stomach's hydrochloric acid, thereby reducing the ability to digest or break down food and thereby being a likely cause of digestive upsets and gastric disturbances. Yet, carbonated minerals are often considered the standard from which to compare other calcium supplements due to their absorbability. However, there is no reason to put up with one type of mineral's undesired effects for its advantages when other types of minerals do not require any sacrifice whatsoever. Often, people mistake the reason for their indigestion is because of excess stomach acid, and then habitually reach for digestive aids containing mineral carbonates and therefore continually perpetuate the problem. Unless you have an ulcer, eating plenty of enzyme-active foods and a good digestive enzyme tablet are what is needed to help digest your foods and eliminate gastric malfunctioning.

Rather than encourage more digestive problems through taking supplements that neutralize stomach acids after a meal, it is more effective for thorough digestion and nutrient absorption to include a digestive enzyme tablet in your supplementation. A daily supplement containing protease and amylase enzymes helps split the dense molecular structures of proteins and carbohydrates, respectively, which helps prevent gastric and intestinal flare-ups. A digestive enzyme supplement should also contain lipase, the enzyme needed for producing bile acids required for digesting fats.

Minerals are too important for protecting your health to chance trying to save money on cheap elemental mineral supplements that are non-absorbable, or on those that hinder digestion and may create inflammatory conditions as the body attempts to eliminate them. Upon examining countless nutritional supplements for over three and a half decades, I have rejected all but just a few of the formulations on the market due to their containing inadequate forms of minerals, *no matter how many otherwise impressive ingredients they contained.* Mineral absorbability should be the first item you zero in on when examining a product's label, and should be the main determining factor in your purchasing decision; they are that important to your health. The small percentage of the manufacturers who obviously do their scientific homework and care enough about their customers to put out an effective product deserve your business, and those who are willing to provide you with answers to your questions satisfactorily and disclose as much information as you might ask for, deserve your trust.

Minerals are the most difficult nutrients to obtain through food since conventional agriculture does not replenish the soils with minerals other than phosphorus and potassium, and the mass production of organically grown food ingredients may not ensure you are getting the full range of known essential minerals either. Absorbable forms of minerals in your multi-nutrient supplement formulation can therefore fulfill any possible mineral deficiencies in your daily dietary intake of even organically grown foods. An effective nutritional supplement is still a wise investment for safeguarding your health even if your food comes from smaller scale farmers growing organic foods who are faithfully replenishing their soil nutrients and doing all they can to maintain a balanced ecosystem and sustainable environment.

Even then, one can never be sure, not without objective laboratory analysis of soil samples disclosed by the farm operation itself, and such information should not be an unreasonable request from any customer. Also, strict FDA regulations on labeling accuracy and operational monitoring should provide reasonable assurance that the end product itself contains what the label says it does. Absorbable minerals are therefore the most critical component in any cost effective and nutritionally effective formulation, and their absorbability the deciding factor in your purchase.

Essential Major Minerals
(Measured in Milligrams)

Sodium - Important component of blood plasma, regulates water uptake into the cell, allows muscles to contract normally, required for normal nervous system functioning, required for digestive process.

Potassium - Assists cells in determining what is allowed inside the cell, assists nerves in sensory cognition, essential for nerve transmission and release of biochemicals in this process, works with sodium to regulate water balance in and outside of the cells.

Calcium - Essential for building strong bones and teeth, controls muscle growth and contractions, helps control electrical impulses to the brain, helps maintain proper blood pressure, helps blood clotting in cuts to stop bleeding, plays a role in digestion and energy production cycles.

Boron - Assists calcium in building strong bones, helps with proper brain functioning, helps increase mental alertness, helps improve attention and short-term memory. Allows calcium, magnesium and phosphorus to function properly.

Magnesium - Involved in energy production, metabolism of carbohydrates and fats, required for forming DNA/RNA. Deficiencies of protein, calcium, zinc and Vitamin D impair absorption of this mineral.

Manganese - Activator of multiple enzymes involved in ATP (adenosine tri-phosphate) synthesis for cell energy production and in metabolism of carbohydrates, amino acids, and cholesterol.

Phosphorus - Required by every cell in the body for normal functioning. Along with calcium, is a major component of bone in the form of phosphate. Needed for cell energy production during the ATP energy cycle and for energy storage. A major component of DNA/RNA, is needed for storing and transmitting genetic information. Required for activating enzymes, hormones and cell-signaling communication. Helps in blood hemoglobin functioning and in delivering oxygen to body tissues.

Zinc - Helps balance blood sugar, helps maintain a healthy immune system, helps provide an optimal sense of smell and taste, helps stabilize rate of metabolism.

Selenium - Antioxidant, protects cells from free radical damage, allows thyroid to produce thyroid hormone, helps reduce risk of joint inflammation.

Sulfur - Besides calcium and phosphorus, sulfur is the third most abundant mineral in the body. Used as a safe and potent medicine for thousands of years, this essential mineral is used in every single cell throughout the entire human body and is so essential to life that we cannot live without it. However, sulfur is often excluded from lists of essential minerals because it is present in all amino acids, the basic foundation of all protein molecular structures in the body.

Sulfur is usually abundant in the average diet, and also in lacto-ovo vegetarian diets and also in vegetarian diets that include fish. Sulfur is plentiful in animal-derived protein foods and many vegetables. Sulfur is a component of vitamin B1 and other biochemicals the body manufacturers. Sulfur is a part of the components of hair, skin, nails and cartilage in bone joints in the form of chondroitin sulfate and glucosamine sulfate, and is present in cartilage in the nose and ears.

Sulfur is important in the detoxification of the blood, liver, glandular system and other organs. Utilizing sulfur, the liver converts an accumulation of fat-soluble, toxic chemicals from the environment and works to convert them to water soluble substances that can more easily be eliminated by the body's eliminative channels: the bowels, kidneys, lungs, lymph circulatory system and skin. Sulfur, along with other plant phytonutrient constituents, has powerful antibacterial properties.

Essential Micro Minerals
(Measured in micrograms)

Copper - Essential in reducing free radicals, preserving cells' electron configurations; involved in strong and flexible connective tissue, essential to brain and nervous system, prevents anemia along with iron.

Chloride - One of the main electrolytes in the body important for working with potassium and sodium in conducting proper electrical impulses in the nervous system. Combines with hydrogen in the stomach to produce hydrochloric acid, the highly acidic digestive enzyme required to break down protein foods. Needed to activate intrinsic factor in order to absorb vitamin B12. Helps control pH balance in the body, helps transport carbon dioxide out of the body during respiration. (Not to be confused with chorine, a deadly gas.)

Iron - Red blood cell oxygen transport and oxygen storage in muscle cells, critical to cell energy production.

Iodine - Glandular-regulating mineral, involves brain hypothalamus and pituitary glands, prevents brain damage.

Chromium - Critical for blood sugar (blood glucose) metabolism. Enhances insulin effects.

Molybdenum - Cofactor-catalyst for enzyme biochemical reactions involving protein metabolism, detoxification and forming new RNA/DNA for new cell genesis.

Using the nutrient evaluation chart below can help you determine adequate potencies when selecting an effective multi-nutrient supplement. This reference chart will help you determine the vitamin-mineral potencies on product labels when selecting vitamin and mineral supplement products. Units of measurements listed are weight measurements in milligrams or micrograms for water-soluble nutrients.

Fat soluble vitamins are measured as international units, listed on product labels as I.U. Supplement manufacturers must follow the FDA's Current Good Manufacturing Practices (CGMP) to ensure labeling data matches what is in the product, that product quality is consistent and quality control is optimal (U.S. Food and Drug 2010).

**RDA (Recommended Daily Allowance)
Versus Optimal and Maximum Safe Intakes For Vitamins**

Vitamins	RDA for Men	RDA for Women*	Optimal Adult Intake	Maximum Safe Intake for Healthy Adults[†††]
Vitamin A	5,000 IU	4,000 IU	10,000 IU	25,000 IU[††]
Thiamin	1.5 mg	1.1 mg to 1.5 mg	100-300 mg	No known limit
Riboflavin	1.7 mg	1.3-1.7 mg	100-300 mg	No known limit
Niacin	19 mg	15-19 mg	50-100 mg[#]	No known limit
Vitamin B6	2.0 mg	1.6-2.0 mg	50-300 mg	500 mg
Folate (folic acid)	200 mcg	180-400 mcg	400 mcg	No known limit
Vitamin B12	2.0 mcg	1.6-2.0 mcg	5-100 mcg	No known limit
Biotin	30-100 mcg**	30-100 mcg**	300 mcg	No known limit
Pantothenic Acid	4-7 mg**	4-7 mg**	10-300 mg	No known limit
Vitamin C	60 mg	60-82 mg	100-2,000 mg[#]	No known limit
Vitamin D	200 IU	200 IU	400 IU	15,000 IU
Vitamin E	15 IU	12-15 IU	200-600 IU	No known limit
Vitamin K	80 mcg**	65 mcg**	100 mcg	500 mcg

RDA (Recommended Daily Allowance)
Versus Optimal and Maximum Safe Intakes For Minerals

Minerals	RDA for Men	RDA for Women*	Optimal Adult Intake	Maximum Safe Intake for Healthy Adults[†††]
Calcium	1.000-1,200 mg	1,200-1,000 mg	1,200 mg[#]	2,500 mg
Chromium	50-200 mcg**	50-200 mcg**	50-200 mcg	200 mcg
Copper	1.5-3.0 mg**	1.5-3.0 mg**	3.0 mg	3.0 mg
Iodine	150 mcg	150-187 mcg	150 mcg	2.0 mg
Iron	10 mg	15-30 mg	18 mg	50-100 mg
Magnesium	350 mg	280-337 mg	600 mg	No known limit
Manganese	2.0-5.0 mg**	2.0- 5.0- mg**	10 mg	No known limit
Molybdenum	75-250 mcg	75-250 mcg	250 mcg	500 mcg
Phosphorus	800 mg	800- 1200 mg	1,200 mg	No known limit
Potassium	2,000 mg[†]	2,000 mg[†]	3,500 mg	15,000 mg
Selenium	70 mcg	55-70 mcg	200 mcg	200 mcg
Zinc	15 mg	12-17 mg	30 mg	500 mg

*RDA range indicates allowances for pregnant and nursing women.

**No RDA but is established as an estimated safe and adequate daily intake.

†No RDA but is an estimated minimum requirement.

††Reflects research showing reduction of disease risk or reduction of risk factors for disease. Pregnant women, women attempting pregnancy, or women at risk of unplanned pregnancy _must not_ exceed the RDAs.

†††Upper limits apply only to healthy adults not pregnant or taking prescription drugs. "No limit," does not mean one can consume more than the Optimal Adult Intake. Any one vitamin or mineral excess can interfere with absorption or uitilization of others and must be taken in proper balance. Exceeding the Optimal Adult Intake produces no benefits; however, nutrient therapy for preventing specific disease conditions must be performed by a qualified health practitioner.

#Intake of levels over the Optimal Adult Intake may produce minor side effects or cause uncomfortable symptoms.

(Fleger 2013)

5 Other Supplements--The Whole Food Synergy Advantage

The full range of known essential vitamins and minerals should be included in every multi-nutrient nutritional supplement. Formulations containing naturally derived vitamins and absorbable forms of minerals provide a solid foundation from which to build and maintain optimal health and to protect the body from an array of deficiency diseases. However, vitamins and minerals are only the framework from which to fill in various other nutritional substances vital to successfully mastering your health.

When putting together your nutritional supplement protocol, it is important to remember the Complete and Correct Supplement Equation Formula:

Naturally-Derived Vitamins + Absorbable Minerals + Whole Food Synergy = Intensified Effectiveness = Greater Health.

Many nutritional supplement formulations contain a variety of unnecessary "Other Ingredients". The typical challenge of selecting any supplement is to prevent redundancy between products ensure adequate potency, avoid non-absorbable or poorly absorbable substances, and reject any formulation containing synthetic and potentially toxic or allergenic ingredients. Already discussed are the types of vitamins and minerals to be preferred in selecting a supplement, which should be the fundamental basis for every nutritional supplementation protocol. The focus on bio-available, whole food or whole food derived ingredients is equally important for your health investment. What follows are supplements that are important additions to one's nutritional supplementation that enhance the effectiveness of vitamins and minerals, and why one selects any of them depends upon a variety of factors which will be discussed in the next sections.

Amino Acids

Foods that provide the body with energy are known as the energy nutrients, and are classified as protein, fats and carbohydrates. These energy nutrients should be consumed in balanced proportions relative to each other for satisfying the body's energy and metabolic requirements and for maintaining all bodily processes. However, skipping meals, hasty meal choices, or being misinformed about how to choose foods for satisfying the body's optimum energy needs often results in imbalanced and nutrient deficiencies. The body needs all eight amino acids present at every meal to meet its protein requirements for the day, and this nutritional requirement can be satisfied most thoroughly and consistently with animal-derived protein foods.

If you are unable or neglect to take in adequate amounts of protein foods on a daily basis, you may want to consider an amino acid supplement to help ensure the continued maintenance and optimal functioning of your entire body's cells, tissues, fluids and structures. If you are recovering from an injury or illness, an amino acid supplement can help fulfill the body's need for the "building blocks of life", providing all eight essential amino acids critically needed to heal and recuperate and with adequate amounts to do the job. If you are focused on progressing toward a higher level of fitness or are a serious athlete regularly challenging your limits, an amino acid supplement becomes a vital, essential-to-life component in your supplementation. Amino acids are vital for perpetuating the ongoing production of biochemicals that perform essential biological processes in all body systems. If you recall, other than being 70% water, the human body is composed mostly of protein.

If one does not have the time nor take the time to prepare biologically correct, nutritionally balanced meals, one or more of energy-providing foods missing or deficient in one's daily food intake results in an energy and nutrient deficit. As a nutritional consultant I have often been surprised at the inconsistent amounts of dietary protein in people's diets while they suffered ailments from protein deficiencies. If one has a habit of not consuming enough protein foods such as meats, poultry, fish, eggs and dairy products, the body's biological processes are often compromised.

If any essential amino acid is missing at any given moment during any biological process, the new biosynthesis of new cell production or the construction of any one of trillions of essential body proteins comes to an immediate halt, and the body is forced to borrow from its own tissues elsewhere by breaking down valuable and much needed body protein. This creates an overall protein deficit and slows down other essential bodily processes, including energy production and immune system defenses. Habitually depriving your body of protein results in a weakened physical condition and diminished overall body protein because it must borrow from less vital yet much needed areas, such as cartilage, blood, bone and muscle to meet its higher priority protein needs.

Enough daily dietary protein must be ingested for daily metabolic processes such as maintaining brain and nerve cells, vital organs, immune cells, and for the manufacture of innumerable enzyme catalysts, regulating and monitoring hormones, critical protein carriers of nutrients and other biochemicals to and from all cells. These critical processes occur 24 hours a day, every day of your life. More energy calories are used to fuel such cellular processes than used to fuel muscles.

Therefore, to ensure you are fulfilling your body's extensive protein requirements, an amino acid supplement may be warranted if you tend to skip meals, are subjecting yourself to many physical challenges in your workout regimen, or are recovering from injury, surgery, or healing other kinds of health conditions in collaboration with your physician. If one is physically active, the more challenging workout sessions can be without replenishing the body adequately with protein and all other nutrients after every session. The more often one pushes the body to meet those challenges, the higher the nutrient and energy calorie requirement is to maintain a desired level of fitness. The better you satisfy your protein/amino acid requirements, the more physical capacity and mental toughness you can maintain to stay in the peak of health or provide the essential materials needed to heal your body.

There are about 28 amino acids that are combined to create the hundreds of proteins that the body needs for life. The body can manufacture all but eight amino acids essential for staying alive and well, and out of these essential eight, the body can manufacture the other twenty. Protein is vital to survival, and each essential amino acid is at the basis of all life metabolic processes. Since all eight essential amino acids are required in substantial amounts to maintain life, and if you tend to neglect your protein needs for whatever reason, it may be critical for you to select an amino acid supplement containing those essential eight. Consuming individual amino acids is futile since they work in concert. Any protein/amino acid deficiencies or imbalances can reduce your overall daily functioning.

The Eight Essential Amino Acids

Choose an amino acid supplement that contains the following eight essential. Some formulations also include the other twenty amino acids, even though, as you know, the body can manufacture them from the essential eight. Some amino acid formulations also contain plant sterols, enzymes and other nutrients, which is fine as long as there are no toxic or potentially allergenic other ingredients. For more information about toxic ingredients, see Chapter Six.

Tryptophan - Helps alleviate insomnia and induces normal sleep. Reduces anxiety and depression. Helps in the treatment of migraine headaches; helps the immune system; helps reduce the risk of artery and heart spasms; works with lysine in reducing cholesterol levels.

Lysine - Insures the adequate absorption of calcium; helps form collagen, which makes up bone cartilage and connective tissue; aids in the production of antibodies, hormones and enzymes. Lysine may be effective against herpes by improving the balance of nutrients that reduce viral growth. A deficiency may result in tiredness, inability to concentrate, irritability, bloodshot eyes, retarded growth, loss of hair, anemia and reproductive problems.

Methionine - Helps supply sulfur which prevents disorders of the hair, skin and nails; helps lower cholesterol levels by increasing the liver's production of lecithin; reduces liver fat and protects the kidneys; a natural chelating agent for heavy metals; regulates the formation of ammonia and creates ammonia-free urine which reduces bladder irritation; influences hair follicles and promotes hair growth.

Phenylalanine - Used by the brain to produce norepinephrine, a chemical that transmits signals between nerve cells and the brain; keeps you awake and alert; reduces hunger pains; functions as an antidepressant and helps improve memory.

Threonine - An important constituent of collagen, elastin, and enamel protein; helps prevent fat build-up in the liver; helps the digestive and intestinal tracts function more smoothly; assists metabolism and assimilation.

Valine - Promotes mental capacity, muscle coordination and calm emotions.

Leucine and **Isoleucine** - Provide ingredients for the manufacturing of other essential biochemical components in the body, some of which are utilized for the production of energy, act as stimulants to the upper brain and promote mental alertness.

Antioxidants

Antioxidants include a variety of vitamins, minerals, enzymes, and phytonutrients found in whole foods and in functional botanicals known as nutraceuticals. These nutrients and naturally occurring biochemical substances found in plants offer powerful protection against scavenging free radicals that typically cause damage to living cells. Free radicals are highly reactive chemicals that occur when a molecule or atom gains or loses a negatively charged electron particle. Although free radicals occur in the body during normal metabolism, high concentrations of exogenous free radicals from chemical pollutants and illness-causing organisms can damage a cell's DNA, prevent the manufacture of new proteins, and damage cell components, including the cell's safeguarding membrane. Such free radical damage to cells is associated with developing various diseases, including cancer.

Antioxidants often possess an abundance of electrons, so are able to donate electrons to free radicals, thereby neutralizing those destructive substances' potentially damaging effects. Antioxidants protect against cell component damage, including the genetic code in the

DNA. Your body attempts detoxification using various elimination channels but is not always successful if the chemical body burden is too overwhelming. Constant daily bombardment from toxic agricultural chemicals, industrial pollutants, and skin and lung exposure to synthetic chemicals found in most personal care, household and industrial products are considered dangerous free radicals that can damage or transpose human genetic code sequencing in the DNA. Once the gene order is disrupted, cells multiplying and replicating in that confused state is where the disease process begins.

The corrective biochemical properties of plant-derived foods or healing botanicals containing antioxidant phytonutrients are also needed if one habitually consumes processed, molecularly distorted foods, such as oils that have undergone hydrogenation or grains that have been refined and partitioned from the whole plant. If one uses nutrient-destructive cooking methods such as high frying temperatures in oil, or eats foods containing GMOs (genetically modified organisms) or toxic chemicals, phytonutrients become extremely important.

GMOs are the result of unregulated biotechnology that includes seeds used in various crops having been transgenically manipulated and engineered with the genetic material of another organism such as an insect or animal, or having been genetically manipulated by inserting a pesticide into a seed's genetic material. This practice has not only resulted in nutrient-devoid, toxic foods, scavenging insects are adapting to the pesticides and are being termed "superbugs" because they are actually adjusting to the toxins. Common weeds are now called "superweeds" as they have also adapted to the increased spraying of herbicides. More and more toxic chemicals are being applied to crops with more damage to the environment upon which all living things depend, including ourselves.

Through such contamination of the environment, major genetic disruptions in all forms of life, including an increased incidence of genetic defects and other serious debilitating diseases now running rampant in human populations, have contributed to adverse, cascading effects on the complex interdependency of ecosystems throughout the world, resulting in increased toxic chemical pollution in the soils and planetary water sources. Consuming pesticide-ridden foods not grown organically is a major threat to human and animal health.

Daily exposure to thousands of chemicals over several decades has increased the amount of toxic chemicals retained in the body tissues and body fluids of each individual, and with each succeeding generation, has put a person at higher risk for the degenerative disease process and more damage to his or her genetic code. Now more than ever in the history of humankind has the reversing of such widespread species and environmental damage been more desperate.

The more people understand the connection between their own less than optimal or declining health and the increased incidence of disease on such an epidemic scale, the more it can be perceived how critical consumer choices are for protecting their health. Increasing one's individual intake of antioxidant phytonutrients can help protect or revive their health through the detoxification, DNA-repairing capacity of those phytonutrients.

By encouraging environmentally conscious businesses that support the sustainable production of safe, nontoxic, nutrient-rich crops, the better one can achieve optimal health with superior nutritional supplements that are truly effective. Although the human body requires a full range of vitamins and minerals to stay alive and thrive, the antioxidant properties of plants containing a great amount of various phytonutrients are critical for your protection and for protecting optimally thriving environments from which your supplements' ingredients are derived. The more informed choices you make with global awareness in mind starting with your own inner universe, the greater our chances of becoming great stewards and caretakers of this beautiful, ancient world.

Although within the body's inner micro-universe it is able to manufacture some antioxidants to neutralize naturally occurring free radicals, it is often overwhelmed by the task of protecting its genetic code due to the toxic chemical body burden from the daily assault of thousands of toxic chemicals that are fat-soluble, and stored in the body's fatty tissues, including the glands, lymph nodes and the brain. Never before has it been more critical to add antioxidant supplementation to your daily nutritional intake to boost your food's detoxifying ability and maintain your health freedom of choice. By supporting all forms of businesses through your own personal consumer selections that protect your health, you help form a formidable consumer force that competes with the deep pockets and influence of mega corporations that are responsible for instilling poor consumer choices that lead to degenerative disease and destruction of whole environments.

The financial success of mega corporate agriculture, chemical, pharma and other mega corporations enable them to influence the media and the education and socialization of the masses, and have integrated their monopolies in order to influence all aspects of your life, including how healthy you are or how diseased you become. However, because of technology, people are now able to distribute information to thousands of others immediately and rapidly enact change.

Because of the growing awareness of the masses of informed citizens, they are actually impacting the behavior of those entities that for decades may have kept you, an amazing human being, from discovering your untapped, true health potential. Because of this growing awareness and access to obscured information, corporate exploitations have been gradually losing their influence and power, as their destructive affronts to life and environment are crumbling under the pressure. New choices of people the world over demanding a more holistic management of health and environment are having a significant impact on the quality of foods and supplements being produced.

An aware and monitoring citizenry required to oversee irresponsible corporate behavior means having optimal mental and physical capabilities optimized through complete and correct nutrition and supplementation. The increase of greater numbers of healthy populations and raising awareness of how to improve one's health potential can eventually outweigh exposure to harmful substances and reduce severe chronic nutrient deficiencies through educated choices.

The types of supplements that must be encouraged are those formulated with a broader holistic perspective, being powerful enhancements for fulfilling individual health needs while contributing to global responsibility. It is now critical that our every choice can make the difference whether the human race and all we affect will continue as it has for thousands of years, or rapidly become extinct. Never in human history has it been more imperative that human beings collectively act on a larger scale to reverse the polluting and devastating effects on the world's interdependent ecologies and global weather.

There are thousands of antioxidant phytochemicals containing essential oils and other constituents in whole, fresh foods and natural medicinals that have been shown to bind to toxic chemicals and help the body eliminate them, and to actually correct confused gene sequencing in the DNA double helix, thereby averting the disease process and protecting your genetic code. In view of the nutritional deficiency disease epidemic that has grown alarmingly throughout humanity in the past fifty years and continues to climb, we can no longer keep neglecting our legacy of the very genetic code that has until now helped us perpetuate ourselves as a robust and thriving species. With each generation that passes, the human genome, our very genetics we pass on to our children, is being severely compromised and degraded. Therefore, anti-oxidant phytonutrients are crucial for the prevention of disease and protecting our very human existence.

Whole food supplements containing anti-oxidant vitamins, minerals and phytonutrients can play a significant role in making the difference between lifelong, vibrant health and disease that is psychologically, emotionally and financially devastating given the high costs of medical care. Considering the thousands of toxins the body is exposed to daily, excluding antioxidants in any nutritional protocol inevitably leads to diseased conditions and premature death.

Purchasing fair trade, organic supplements with potent antioxidant ingredients not only have an important role in boosting the immune system and improving mental functioning and the body's healing capacity, it supports the heroic efforts and dedication of food producers throughout the world that continue to provide you with food and product choices to help fight against diseases associated with chemical toxicity and nutrient deficiencies. Our attention, therefore, is to focus on the most effective supplements you can find. Using the guidelines that follow will provide the information you need to make highly informed nutritional supplement choices and avoid selecting potentially toxic supplements or those with inadequate potencies, poor absorbability or imbalanced formulations.

"Antioxidant" is a general classification that includes certain vitamins, minerals, and plant constituents that protect the body from the disease process and premature aging. It is important to know how much to take of any particular nutrient, and to realize that nutrients function properly when they are present together, for the cascading effect of your body's biochemical processes rely on their cooperative and synergistic functions.

Below is a chart listing vitamins and minerals that have antioxidant properties, although government guidelines for nutrients still do not distinguish between synthetic and naturally derived vitamins and minerals.

Vitamin and Mineral Antioxidants

Vitamin	Government RDA	Optimal Adult Intake	Maximum Safe Intake
Vitamin C	75-90 mg	100-2,000 mg	No known limit
Vitamin E (mixed tocopherols)	15 I.U.	200-600 mg	No known limit
Mineral	**Government RDA**	**Optimal Adult Intake**	**Maximum Safe Intake**
Selenium	55 mcg	200 mcg	200 mcg
Zinc	8-12 mg	40 mg	40 mg

Reference sources: ("Dietary Supplement Fact Sheet 2013), (Vitamin C 2013), (Fleger 2013)

Phytonutrient Antioxidants

Carotenoids – There are over 600 natural pigments that occur in fruits and vegetables, and are what give them their yellow, orange and red colors. The most common dietary carotenoids can be divided into two classes: the carotenes and the xanthophylls. The carotenes are alpha-carotene, beta-carotene and beta-cryptoxanthin, and the xanthophylls are lutein, lycopene, and zeaxanthin.
The body is able to convert carotenes to retinol, a form of vitamin A when needed, and therefore do not pose a

risk of overdose and toxicity as vitamin A supplements derived from fish oils do, or as does synthetic vitamin A. A minimum of 3-5 grams of dietary fat from whole food sources allows higher absorption and utilization of carotenoids. The body can store large amounts of carotene in its fatty tissues without any known toxicity; however, the skin can take on an orange color when tissues become more saturated. Ceasing or reducing carotene supplemental dosages allows the body time to gradually utilize or eliminate the excess.

Studies reveal that isolated beta-carotene supplements may increase the risk of lung cancer in smokers and former asbestos workers, and although beta-carotene supplements do not reduce the risk of cardiovascular disease, whole food sources containing several carotenoids reduce the risk of heart disease and cancer. Therefore, when choosing a supplement that helps fulfill the body's vitamin A requirements, a supplement containing a variety of carotenoids from whole foods is the wiser choice, rather than supplements consisting of only beta-carotene or only vitamin A.

The xanthophylls are not converted to retinol (vitamin A) and therefore are not involved in vitamin A activity, but are potent antioxidants nonetheless. The xanthophylls lutein and zeaxanthin are carotenoids found in the eye's retina and lens, and research indicates they may slow macular degeneration due to aging, and help prevent cataracts. Epidemiological studies found that men less likely to develop prostate cancer consumed lycopene from tomatoes and tomato products compared to those who did not consume those foods (Higdon 2009).

Chlorophyll – A photoreceptor molecule in plants that absorbs sunlight and uses the energy to synthesize carbohydrates and water during the process of photosynthesis, and it is the stored energy in chlorophyll that sustains the plant's life processes. Chlorophyll is the pigment that gives plants their green color, and since it is molecularly very similar to red blood cells, it is highly bio-available and absorbable. Chlorophyll is able to bind to chemicals known to cause cancer, particularly polycyclic aromatic hydrocarbons from tobacco smoke, heterocyclic amines in cooked meat, and aflatoxin-B1. Chlorophyll binds to cancer-causing chemicals and interferes with their absorption in the gastrointestinal tract, and seems able to neutralize free radicals that cause oxidative damage, including free radicals generated by radiation therapy (Chlorophyll 2009)

Isothiocyanates - This class of sulfur containing compounds found in cruciferous vegetables such as broccoli, cauliflower, Brussels sprouts, cabbage, kale, bok choy, turnip, kohlrabi, turnips and water cress are released during the process of chewing or when these vegetables are cut up, and are much more potent when they are raw, for they lose 60% of their effectiveness when cooked. The addition of vegetables and greens containing Isothiocyanates make excellent additions to supplement formulations, especially if their active enzymes are not destroyed.

Isothiocyanates play an important role in helping the body eliminate carcinogens or cancer-causing substances, drugs, and many toxins. Isothiocyanates also protect the normal cell cycle of division and replication, where it is determined whether a cell's DNA can be repaired or destroyed through pathways leading to programmed cell death (apoptosis). When cell regulation processes go wrong, it may result in the propagation of mutations leading to cancer, but isothiocyanates can inhibit the proliferation of cancer cells and help induce cancer cell apoptosis. Isothiocyanates also possess anti-inflammatory activity that prevents the development of cancer, and shows some antibacterial activity against the bacteria H. pylori, which is associated with an increased risk of gastric cancer (Higdon 2005).

Phytosterols - Similar in molecular structure to cholesterol, these compounds assist in recirculating cholesterol for its improved use and elimination of it out of the body when necessary. Since phytosterols can only be absorbed in trace amounts, they help reduce absorption of intestinal cholesterol, which leads to decreased blood LDL "bad" cholesterol levels, lowering the risk for cardiovascular disease. Research shows that phytosterols act in several ways to inhibit cancer cell proliferation and are involved in self-destruction or apoptosis of cancer cells. Phytosterols indicate an ability to increase antioxidant enzyme activity and therefore reduce oxidation or formation of free radicals (Woyengo 2009).

Phytosterols are added to some processed foods because they can be dispersed in water when emulsified with lecithin. and reduce cholesterol absorption by competing with cholesterol for absorption in the digestive tract. Phytosterols are not themselves easily absorbed, further helping to lower blood cholesterol. Dietary intakes vary from 167-437 mg/day and up to 2000 mg or 2 g per day are considered safe supplemental doses. There are over 200 known phytosterols, according to the National Institutes of

Health, and can be derived from greens and other vegetables, plant oils from nuts and seeds, whole grains, spices and their seeds. A well-thought out formulation that includes whole food phytosterols, which are high in antioxidants, is definitely one to consider in your nutritional supplement choices since scientific studies indicate they are a good preventive measure against stroke, heart disease, and breast, lung, ovarian and stomach cancer (Bano 2013).

Phytosterols help stop the slowed production of collagen that occurs as the body ages, and supports the production of new collagen, providing a firmer, more flexible and youthful skin structure. Collagen is the main component of connective tissue in the skin, and the aging process reduces the amount of collagen the body produces, resulting in sagging skin. Phytosterols improve the skin's composition by helping to improve its connective tissue structure. Phytosterols also help improve immune system functioning through their direct activity in protecting the body's lymph system, and have been used in therapies where chronic inflammatory conditions occur when treating cardiovascular disease and cancer.

A scientific review of therapeutic levels of phytosterols revealed that the amount of fat-soluble vitamin A in the blood was not affected by consuming large amounts of phytosterols. Vitamin D was apparently not affected or lowered slightly, vitamin E was lowered, vitamin K was reduced by 14 percent, and blood level carotenoids reduced by 10-20 percent. Higher doses of any one isolated nutritional component usually affects other nutritional factors due to the imbalances it can create, and may result in undesirable side effects such as diarrhea, vomiting, stomach cramping, nausea, and skin, nasal, eye or throat irritation. Nutrients and plant components work best in synergy; it is therefore always wise to stick to the recommended safe known ranges and choose phytosterol supplements containing whole food ingredients (Bano 2013).

Lycopene - One of the carotenoids the body is able to convert to vitamin A as needed, and is a naturally occurring pigment that gives red, yellow and orange fruits and vegetables their bright colors. As a powerful antioxidant, it has a neutralizing effect on scavenging free radicals that aggressively cause oxidative damage in cells and their functioning. Lycopene is associated with reduced incidence of certain cancers and protects against stroke, along with a lowered risk of heart attack or myocardial infarction (Godman 2012). Typical lycopene supplement dosages are 2-30 milligrams, and are extracted from tomatoes, watermelon, or pink or red grapefruit.

Proanthocyanidins – This group of antioxidant phytochemicals (plant chemicals) is found mainly in grape skins and seeds, and is also present in red wine due to the fermentation process where the proanthocyanidins are extracted through the formed alcohol. Proanthocyanidins are important in preventing the formation of free radicals during normal metabolic functions, have been shown to be anti-carcinogenic, anti-tumoral and anti-allergenic by inhibiting the production of histamine, help prevent cardiovascular disease through improving cholesterol HDL/LDL ratios and blood pressure, improve fat metabolism as well as help reduce atherosclerosis. Proanthocyanidins have also been shown to protect the heart against damage from inhaled aerosol asthma treatments ("Proanthocyanidins" n.d.).

Resveratrol – A flavonol and part of a group of flavonoids that plants produce to protect them against disease. Resveratrol is found in blueberries, eucalyptus, mulberries, peanuts, red grapes, red wine and spruce. Higher resveratrol content in wines depends on how long it undergoes fermentation. Resveratrol has been shown to have anti-cancer properties, prevents damage caused by cholesterol LDL, the heavy metal cadmium, UV radiation and nitrite radicals. Resveratrol protects against DNA damage, including cancer or the formation of tumors by inhibiting cyclo-oxygenase-1, an enzyme that converts arachidonic acid to tumor promoting substances. It has also been indicated that resveratrol may protect cells from damage caused by high blood sugar levels (blood glucose), and helps reduce neuropathic (nerve) pain. An effective antioxidant, resveratrol is a good free radical scavenger, protects against the oxidation of lipids and protects endothelial cells from free radical damage. It also helps prevent heart damage after cardiac arrest and reduces risk of platelet aggregation leading to atherosclerosis (Resveratrol n.d.).

Xanthones – found in the mangosteen fruit rind or pericarp, xanthones are a class of potent antioxidants with many beneficial pan-systemic effects on the body. Studies show that xanthones are antitumoral, antiallergenic, anti-inflammatory, antibacterial, anti-fungal, and antiviral. The mangosteen fruit pericarp has traditionally been applied by indigenous healers and used in medical systems outside of Western medicine to and for patients suffering from fever, infection, dysentery and digestive disorders (Xanthones, Food Chem Toxicol 2008).

Other Antioxidants

Coenzyme Q10 - A compound made naturally in the body that helps cells produce energy, is instrumental during their growth and protects them against free radical damage. CoQ10, also known as ubiquinone or ubidecarenone, is found mostly in the heart, liver, kidneys and pancreas. Low blood levels of CoQ10 are present in myeloma and lymphoma patients, and those with breast, colon, kidney, lung, head and neck cancer ("Questions and Answers About Coenzyme Q10"2013).

Research concludes CoQ10 is beneficial for maintaining normal blood pressure and cholesterol, protecting DNA or genetic material, and contributes to normal cognitive functioning. CoQ10 is best absorbed when taken with dietary fats; lipid preparations are therefore better absorbed than the purified compound (EFSA 2010).

Clinical research demonstrates CoQ10's effectiveness for prolonging exercise performance in healthy individuals in aerobic power, anaerobic threshold and more rapid heart rate and volume oxygen recovery, but only within the limits of the ability of cells to uptake and utilize it (Cooke March 4, 2008).

For adults 19 years and older, the recommended dosages are 30-200 mg daily. Caution should be used if taking medications; it is best to check with your medical provider to ensure CoQ10 does not interfere with the intended effects of any prescribed drugs. No formal scientific studies has shown that CoQ10 results in any adverse side effects other than a few reports of stomach upset, but it has not been determined if this supplement should be taken while pregnant or breastfeeding. Since CoQ10 may lower blood sugar, diabetics should check with their physician before taking it ("CoEnzyme Q10" 2011).

Glutathione - Produced in the liver, is used in chemical reactions and converting nutrients into components within living cells. A key factor for an efficient immune response, glutathione is a protein composed of three amino acids: cysteine, glutamic acid and glyceine. A potent antioxidant, it contributes to the metabolism of nutrients through new protein synthesis, cell proliferation, old or damaged cells' self-destruction or apoptosis, and is involved in cell signaling intracellular communication and the proper expression of genetic material within the DNA. Glutathione is present with high activity in the lungs and other organs and tissues, and high blood levels, particularly among the elderly, are associated with a higher level of health.

Glutathione deficiency is indicated by oxidative stress or vulnerability to free radicals, and therefore leads to more rapid aging and a higher susceptibility to acquiring diseases such as AIDS, Alzheimer's disease, cancer, cystic fibrosis, diabetes, heart disease, HIV, kwashiorkor, liver disease, Parkinson's disease, seizures, sickle cell anemia, and stroke.

Reported medical uses for glutathione supplements include detoxification from heavy metals and the chemotherapy drug *cis-platinum*, treatment of pulmonary fibrosis, Parkinson's disease, reducing blood pressure in diabetics, increasing male sperm count, and treating liver cancer and sickle cell anemia. Currently, scientific literature asserts that ingested glutathione has a negligible effect on how much is transferred inside the cells. It is therefore prudent to provide a full range nutrient supplementation protocol, along with a balanced, nutrient-dense whole food intake to help ensure all necessary factors are present in order for the body to produce its own glutathione (Wu 2004).

Extracts of organosulfur compounds (found in garlic) - Studies on the biological activities of organosulfur compounds found in garlic include inhibiting excess cholesterol formed in the liver, inhibiting abnormal platelet aggregation or blood clotting, inhibiting inflammatory enzymes such as cyclo-oxygenase 2 and lipoxygenase, and inhibiting the formation of atherosclerotic plaques in heart disease. Garlic compounds are converted into hydrogen sulfide by red blood cells to help mediate the need to dilate blood vessels.

Organosulfur compounds inhibit enzymes in the body that activate the cancer forming process while activating enzymes that inhibit potential carcinogens or cancer causing substances. Organosulfur compounds such as that found in garlic may increase production and concentrations of the antioxidant glutathione within cells. Cell culture studies show that organosulfur compounds can arrest the unregulated cell replication of cancerous cells. When cells cannot stop the formation of cancer cell replication because they can no longer be recognized as damaged genetic material, organosulfur compounds are able to induce cell apoptosis, or the self-destruction of replicating cancer cells.

Thiosulfinates, including the garlic extract allicin, are potent anti-bacterial, anti-fungal compounds. In randomized controlled studies, it was found that garlic supplements containing organosulfur compounds helped reduce total serum cholesterol, LDL or "bad" cholesterol, and triglyceride levels by 6-11%.

Note: although garlic extracts show much evidence as effective supplementation for helping to prevent certain diseases, other studies show that whole garlic containing large amounts of organosulfur compounds is more effective in supporting the healing of gastric (stomach) and colorectal cancer. Other studies showed that an increased whole garlic intake reduced the size and number of colorectal polyps, also known as adenomas (Garlic 2013).

Enzymes - The Catalysts of Life

Enzymes, protein biocatalysts generated by cells of humans, plants, or bacteria are key to igniting all biochemical processes. Without enzymes, all biochemical reactions would occur too slowly, if at all, to sustain life. There are metabolic, digestive, and plant enzymes, all of which are critical for the body to use in all bodily processes. Metabolic enzymes are energized protein molecules the body assembles that are needed for food digestion, brain stimulation, cellular energy and repair, and assist in eliminating cellular waste products. The human body assembles, disassembles and reassembles vast numbers of vital-to-life metabolic enzymes, and only does so to the extent of the completeness of nutrients and dietary enzymes a person eats.

Dietary enzymes are obtained through enzyme-active, fresh foods and may be contained in some nutritional supplement formulations. Dietary enzymes along with metabolic enzyme actions during digestion release essential nutrients from food that are needed to sustain life, and provide the precursors for the body's capacity to produce other metabolic enzymes that keep you alive and thriving. Dietary enzymes that are active in fresh foods and preserved in supplements provide the enzymes that aid in breaking down and digesting food down to its most basic components: vitamins, minerals, amino acids from protein foods, fatty acids from fats, and glucose (blood sugar) units of carbon, hydrogen and oxygen from carbohydrates.

From these basic food components, with the aid of enzymes, the body is able to build renewed body proteins, sugars and lipids that make up the entire body's fluids, tissues and structures. Active dietary enzymes are the proteins needed for forming metabolic enzymes necessary for activating and perpetuating all biological processes. A shortage of dietary enzymes could mean a chronic deficiency in the precursors needed to manufacture metabolic enzymes. Therefore, the body's manufacture of metabolic enzymes is dependent on dietary enzymes and augmenting nutrients, and their shortage can result in the halting of any important cellular or biochemical process, and lead to any number of degenerative health conditions or systems malfunctioning.

Through an abundance of dietary enzymes, the body can preserve its ability to generate more metabolic enzymes, including important digestive enzymes amylase, lipase, protease, and lactase, needed to digest various protein, fats and carbohydrate foods.

Digestive Enzymes Produced by the Body

Digestive Enzyme	What They Digest or Break Down
Amylase	Complex carbohydrates (starchy vegetables, grains, legumes)
Lipase	Fats and oils (animal fats, oils in nuts, seeds and some fruits)
Protease	Protein (meats, poultry, fish, eggs, dairy)
Trypsin, Pepsin, Chymotrypsin	Protein
Lactase	Lactose (milk carbohydrate)

Since raw, fresh, enzyme-active foods and enzyme-active supplements are subject to degeneration, foods must be stored properly under refrigeration and supplements kept in airtight product containers. Enzymes are easily destroyed by heat temperatures of over 120 degrees Fahrenheit, by chemical food processing such as pasteurization, sterilization, freezing and microwaving, and overexposure to light and air. Once an enzyme-active food is disconnected from its parent plant and soil nutrient source, its own enzymes serve to break down its fiber and tissue structure toward its own decomposition, so it is better to consume enzyme active foods that are properly ripened and freshly picked, and properly preserved in a nutritional supplement.

Chemical fertilizers, herbicides and pesticides also reduce the amounts of active enzymes in live, fresh foods and may end up in your enzyme-active nutritional

supplement. The green USDA organic seal on the product label assures that no toxic or synthetic chemicals were used in the growing of those food ingredients. A black and white USDA organic seal indicates that only 70% of the ingredients in a product contains organically grown ingredients.
To keep disease-causing chemicals out of your supplements, purchasing products containing organically, sustainably grown ingredients in your supplements not only is an effective health-protective measure, it helps ensure that the organic food production industry can keep growing stronger and continue to help protect a food abundance environment.

Digestive enzymes are found in digestive aid supplement tablets, and some are in chewable form flavored with fruit juices. Digestive enzymes, along with natural food enzymes such as bromelain from pineapples or papain from papaya, can be found in multi-nutrient supplements and fruit-greens-vegetable powders that may also include nut powders and other enzyme-active ingredients. Supplements made with whole food ingredients, particularly when enzymes are preserved and contain fat-soluble vitamins and plant-derived oils, should be kept in airtight containers and refrigerated to prevent the degradation of nutrient quality and exposing their susceptibility to free radical damage, as discussed in the "Antioxidants" section.

The Serrapeptase Enzyme

A third type of enzyme not discussed so far is a systemic proteolytic enzyme known as serrapeptase, which has been shown to be a safe and effective cyclo-oxygenase 2 inhibitor (COX 2 inhibitor) in reducing instances of the body's malfunctioning inflammatory response and therefore reducing pain. Serrapeptase also has been shown to reduce swelling and improve microcirculation, and therefore improves nutrient delivery and oxygenation for more rapid healing. Used in Europe and Asia for over twenty-five years, serrapeptase has been shown to be effective for eliminating toxic cellular metabolic waste products and digestive waste materials, safely reducing the amount of fibrin that forms obstructive clots in the circulatory system, and safely dissolving hardened plaques in the arteries.

Clinical research applying serrapeptase has also shown to induce cancer cell apoptosis (self-destruction) and reduce swelling in fibrocystic breast disease. It also has been shown to safely dissolve atherosclerotic plaques and scar tissue at the micro level, reduce pain of arthritis, help reduce infection in sinusitis, bronchitis and inflammation in other cardiovascular problems.

After discovery and scientific analysis revealed that the pansystemic serrapeptase enzyme had many beneficial properties that could be applied clinically, it has been applied successfully as an aid for pain relief, digestion and a variety of health-improvement applications. Serrapeptase has no typical adverse side effects and hazards of pain reliever medications such as over-the-counter non-steroidal anti-inflammatory drugs (NSAIDS) acetaminophen, ibuprofen or aspirin. NSAIDS come with side effect warnings, cautioning a person seeking pain relief for their possible damage to kidneys, digestive system, and symptoms such as nausea, dizziness, difficulty breathing or swallowing, "swelling of the face, throat, tongue, lips, eyes, hands, feet, ankles, or lower legs", and hives, itching, or rash (Acetaminophen 2013). Or, in the case of aspirin, side effect symptoms include bloody stools, bloody vomit, fast heartbeat and fast breathing, cold clammy skin and ringing of the ears, to name a few (Aspirin 2013). Serrapeptase when used as a pain reliever has no such effects.

Neither a metabolic enzyme produced by the human body nor a food-derived enzyme, serrapeptase is actually derived from a nonpathogenic or non-illness causing intestinal bacteria found in the silkworm. After the silkworm's metamorphosis into a moth, it is able to create an area of escape through its protective cocoon walls composed of silk fibers, one of the strongest natural fibers found in nature. Scientific analysis as to why it is able to accomplish this feat reveals that the serratiopeptidase enzyme produced by the bacterium Serratia marcescens present during the silkworm's regurgitation and exit process actually dissolves the cocoon's tough fibrous material. For production of serrapeptase supplements, the Serratia marcescens bacteria is extracted from the silkworm's intestine and grown in highly selective nutrient culture mediums, where the serratiopeptidase enzyme is recovered and undergoes various types of filtration, purification and characterization for maintaining the quality, value and efficacy of the enzyme (Mohankumar 2011).

As with any supplement, side effects can occur with overuse and inattention to recommended dosing as instructed on product labeling. Cautions against taking serrapeptase include patients who have blood coagulation abnormalities or are taking anti-coagulant medications, or have a liver or kidney disorder. Taking serrapeptase for extended periods or taking it in excess may result in gastrointestinal disturbances, discomfort or nausea, anorexia, or eruption. Lactating, breastfeeding or pregnant women are also cautioned against taking serrapeptase. Since it is a very potent enzyme, literature indicates that long term use is not recommended to prevent the long term use side effects discussed above.

Daily care and attention to eating whole foods with a healthy amount of dietary fiber, regular exercise habits, drinking plenty of clean water, and taking a full range of nutrients and phytonutrients in your supplements leave serrapeptase's role as a temporary measure for healing and restoring the body to its normal balance or homeostasis when needed. If you are suffering from any kind of illness or health abnormality, it would be wise to discuss the use of serrapeptase with your physician, especially if he or she is willing to examine the respectable amount of scientific literature available.

To prevent the degradation of the serratiopeptidase enzyme that would occur in the stomach's gastric hydrochloric acid or digestive juices, serrapeptase tablets are enterically coated in order to reach the higher acidic environment in the small intestine, where it can be slowly absorbed and utilized. When looking for a more effectively absorbed serrapeptase supplement, the enteric coating is key. The composition of enteric coatings vary throughout the supplement and pharmaceutical industries from plant-derived substances to plastic or lacquered coatings. The thicker the coating and farther removed from your body's natural metabolic, digestive enzyme capability, the least likely your serrapeptase tablet may be utilized at all.

Therefore, to ensure your serrapeptase supplement arrives both mostly intact at your intestines and gets absorbed properly, industry labeling recommendations are to take it on an empty stomach, either one half hour before a meal or at least two hours after a meal, and it also makes sense to choose a tablet that is enterically coated with a vegetable coating. However, unless you call the manufacturer and ask, or unless the product label or advertising literature claims the product has a vegetarian coating, you won't know if your product choice will be effective.

Typical serrapeptase supplement potencies are expressed in milligrams per 10,000 units of enzyme activity, such as 5 mg of serrapeptase per 10,000 units, 10 mg of serrapeptase per 20,000 units, 20 mg per 40,000 units, and 30 mg per 60,000 units. Doses range from one to two tablets per day or as recommended on product labeling.

Organic Green Food Powders

Organic green food powders contain a variety of ingredients, and are produced with proprietary manufacturing methods that retain their vitamins, minerals and plant enzymes. Green food powders typically consist of various combinations of ingredients that can help supplement the daily diet:
Algae - chlorella and spirulina

Beans - cacao, carob

Beans, sprouted - adzuki, garbanzo, lentil, kidney

Enzymes - amylase, beta gluconase, cellulase, hemi-cellulase, lipase, papain, pectinase, peptidase, phytase

Fruits and berries - acai, blackberry, blueberry, cherry, raspberry, strawberry, apple, banana, pear, peach, apricot, cucumber, peppers, squash, tomato

Leafy greens - spinach, kale, mustard greens

Grains, sprouted - amaranth, brown rice, buckwheat, millet, quinoa

Grasses - alfalfa, barley, kamut, oat and wheat grass

Herbs - parsley, thyme, onion, chive, garlic bulb

Probiotics - bifidobacterium bifidum, bifidobacterium breve, bifidobacterium lactis, bifidobacterium longum, lactobacillus acidophilus, lactobacillus casei, lactobacillus paracasei, lactobacillus plantarum, lactobacillus rhamnosus, lactobacillus salivarius

Sea vegetables - kelp , dulse

Seeds, sprouted - flax, sunflower, pumpkin,chia, sesame

Spices - ginger

Nut meal - almonds, walnuts

Mushrooms - shitake, mitake

Sweeteners - stevia leaf

Vegetables - asparagus, beets, Brussels sprouts, carrots, broccoli, cauliflower celery, cabbage

These concentrated forms of nutrient dense food ingredients contain a large array of antioxidant phytonutrients, making them an excellent addition to a nutritional supplement protocol for daily detoxification and protection against environmental toxins, as well as for optimizing the body's energy production and nutrient absorption.

Other Whole Food Supplements

Bee pollen - Gathered from flowers, bees ingest pollen to support their nutritional requirements necessary for their development and survival. Pollen is rich in proteins, amino acids, lipids, starch, sterols, vitamins A, B complex, C, D, E and K, bioflavonoids and minerals. Bee pollen has been shown to increase red blood cells and improve oxygen delivery in hemoglobin, be an effective antioxidant for protecting the liver from free radical peroxidation, and to protect the brain from harmful ionizing radiation (Bruno, 2005).

Bee propolis - A resinous substance collected from plants by bees and used in the construction of the beehive. It consists of essential oils, resin and waxes, and amino acids, minerals, vitamins A, B complex, E, flavonoids, and ethanol. Bee propolis has been shown to have anti-fungal, anti-bacterial and anti-viral properties, and helps prevent dental caries (Bruno, 2005).

Royal jelly - Produced by worker honeybees from pollen gathered from flowers, it is secreted by their mandibular and hypopharyngeal glands,and is used to nourish larvae, drones and older workers. The queen bee is fed exclusively the royal jelly, which contains vitamins, minerals, amino acids, lipids and sugars. Royal jelly is what extends the life span of the queen bee, and is how she acquires well-developed gonads. Royal jelly has long been used by people as an anti-aging and fertility supplement. Scientific studies show that RJ contains anti-tumor, antioxidant, anti-inflammatory, anti-bacterial, anti-allergenic, anti-hypertensive, and reduces LDL and total serum cholesterol levels (Hiroyuki, 2012).

Historically, bee pollen, propolis, royal jelly have been considered as valuable nutritional whole food supplements. What makes the valuable food honeybees have always provided to human beings and animals potentially toxic, however, is the increasing amounts of agricultural chemicals affecting the health of bees and other pollinating insects. In the last few decades, the increased use of pesticides on crops has resulted in bee colony collapse disorder, severely reducing bee populations throughout the world. In one study, pesticides, fungicides and herbicides measured in apple, blueberry, cranberry, pumpkin and watermelon crops exceeded the median lethal dose required to kill half a bee population within 24 to 48 hours (Pettis, 2013). If this trend continues, with a major reduction in bee populations, over 50% of our food supply would no longer be available, as without pollination, fruit, nut and other flowering plants would no longer thrive.

Various pesticides have been found in honey at levels that damage the nervous system, disrupt hormones and impair physical development. These neurotoxins are also carcinogenic or cause cancer. The USDA pesticide data program found that when bees roamed in regions without pesticides and brought back to the hives pollen from flowers that were minimally exposed, pesticide levels measured were significantly lower. Pesticide levels in organic honey measured at .2 micrograms per 3.5 ounces, versus .8 micrograms per 3.5 ounces of honey produced from flower pollens exposed to pesticides (Pesticide 2010).

With safety levels measured in parts per billion, sadly, even organic honey's level of pesticides may be putting the health of humans and animals at risk. What you can do as an individual to help reverse this as soon as possible is to focus on organic foods and organic supplement ingredients and therefore supporting the organic food and supplements industries. The greater the demand for organically grown foods, the less it will be profitable for corporations pushing deadly chemicals onto conventional farmers who fear they have no other choice, and the more encouraged farmers become to convert to sustainable organic food production.

Herbs

Herbs are culinary delights that can alter the taste of a meal in many different ways, but they are also powerful foods containing effective phytonutrients that are anti-bacterial, anti-viral, anti-parasitic, and anti-fungal. The phytonutrients in herbs are also able to repair damaged genetic code sequencing in the cell DNA, and can bind to synthetic chemicals to help the body effectively detoxify from harmful pollutants. Herbs, therefore, are also a valuable addition to any supplementation protocol.

There are also thousands of stronger medicinal plants that fall into the category description of an "herb", and have been applied in other medical systems other than Western medicine ,and have been used by indigenous healers throughout the world for thousands of years. The world's healing botanicals, therefore, are best treated with respect, and used under the guidance of a qualified herbalist who understands the scientific evidence confirming their efficacy and appropriate use. All parts of a plant can be considered an herb and each part (e.g., the leaves, flowers or roots) may have a different use.

It is important to familiarize yourself with the beneficial properties of herbs and learn the scientific research available to consumers through valid educational resources from a university (Davis, 2013). This way, you bypass all the marketing and sales hype and confusing dogma circulating around companies interested in selling you their products. There are strict USDA guidelines that prohibit supplement companies from making any medical claims about their products. Organizations such as the Herb Research Foundation and the American Botanical Council are also good resources to obtain reliable information on the beneficial health properties of herbs.

Useful plants are best integrated into your supplemental protocol guided by a qualified herbalist who has examined extensively the scientific literature about herbs' restorative properties. Even then, it's also advocated that you inform your physician if your are under medical care to avoid any possible unwanted side effects or disrupted functioning of your medications.

Scientific studies reveal, however, that herbal therapies applied by medical practitioners around the world are safe and in many cases, more effective than pharmaceutical drugs, and without their harmful side effects. It is recognized that most of the unsubstantiated information on the internet against herbs effectiveness and safety is dogma fueled by the multibillion dollar pharmaceutical and medical business of disease care. Other than forty reported cases of people who have died from the misuse of the Chinese herb ephedra, which has been used successfully in Chinese herbal medicine formulas for thousands of years, it does not compare with the many more thousands of cases of adverse prescription drug reactions that cause deaths every year.

Given the well documented evidence attesting to the safety of herbal remedies compared to the dangers of prescription drugs, it is also well documented that properly prescribed drugs cause thousands of death every year. Regulatory agencies associated with the pharmaceutical industry try to convince the public that it is herbs that are the health threat, when indeed, holistic healers have been quietly healing their clients in spite of the disruptive health dangers of prescription drugs (Gueye, 2011).

Carolyn Dean, M.D., N.D., et. al., conducted an intensive, thorough review of medical, peer-reviewed, scientific journals and government health statistics. In their abstract,"Death by Medicine", they show compelling evidence revealing how much American medicine does more harm than good. It appears that there are entities that are seeking to abolish consumer access to natural therapies and are taking much action any way they can to misinform the public. Here are some facts:

- In 2001 the total number of deaths caused by conventional medicine was 783,936, making the American medical system the leading cause of deaths per year and cost $282 billion.
- The number of deaths from heart disease came in second at 699,697, and the number of deaths from cancer was 553,251.
- Adverse drug reactions causing death were estimated at 106,000, costing $12 billion.
- Medical errors caused 98,000 deaths and the cost was $2 billion.
- Bedsores caused 115,000 deaths and cost $55 billion.
- Infections caused the deaths of 88,000 individuals and cost $5 billion.
- Deaths due to malnutrition were 108,800 at an undetermined cost.
- There were 199,000 outpatient deaths at a cost of $77 billion.
- The 37,136 unnecessary procedures that resulted in deaths cost $122 billion.
- There were 32,000 surgery-related deaths at a cost of $9 billion.
- More than half of the U.S. population, 164 million people, receive unnecessary medical treatment over a ten year span that may lead to death.
- The estimated projected death rates from medical intervention for the next ten years was estimated to be 7,841,360 people, which is reportedly more casualties than all wars fought by Americans in U.S. history.

(Gueye, 2011)

In selecting herbal supplements, consult an herbal database provided by universities, such as North Carolina State University or the University of Maryland. In addition to the HRF and the ABC mentioned above, you can also contact consumer advocate organizations or visit their online databases such as the Linus Pauling Institute at Oregon State University and the Rodale Institute. These educational institutions and organizations are dedicated to preserving herbal knowledge and information about nutrients, organic farming and more.

Consulting a Traditional Chinese Medicine practitioner, a qualified naturopath or holistic nutritionist who is well studied in the scientific literature is also a wise decision when selecting herbs for improving your health. Letting your holistic minded physician know about any herbs you decide to take would be wise, especially if he or she is willing to examine the scientific data of the properties of herbs and how they have been applied clinically in other medical systems of the world, and who will work with you in your herbal selections.

Since herbs are not regulated by the Food and Drug Administration and are classified neither as foods or drugs, the FDA does not monitor the potency of herbal products. Since the administering of herbs is absent in medical training in Western medicine, it is therefore important to learn where the manufacturer obtains a product's ingredients, and learn about the entire production process, starting from the environment in which the raw materials are grown to the end product.

Herbs can be purchased fresh or fresh dried in bulk or in dried powdered form, in capsules or tablet form, in an alcohol based tincture or in a non-alcohol vinegar or vegetable glycerine base. Some food products may contain herbs, or can be purchased as culinary mixtures based on various cultural cuisines. Herbs can also be purchased as herbal extracts, where only one or a few of an herb's medicinal value is partitioned off from the rest of its beneficial substances, which can have a very different effect than the synergistic value and built-in safety of the whole herb. Herbs may also be found in green drinks or in powdered multi-nutrient and whole food supplements and naturopathic remedies. Many savory herbs used in medical systems throughout the world outside of Western medicine are listed in the table below.

Traditional and European, Asian, Indian and other Cultures' Medicinal Uses of Savory Herbs

Herb	Applications
Basil	Used against colds, diarrhea, kidney disease.
Bay (Laurel)	Used for rheumatism, as an embrocation fluid for rubbing on the body for pain relief.
Caper	Astringent, diuretic, expectorant.
Celery	Diuretic, hastens menstrual flow or stimulates blood flow to the pelvic area and uterus (emmenagogue).
Chervil	Diuretic, expectorant, used in beverages as part of a refreshing, invigorating, restorative agent (tonic).
Chive	Antiseptic, diuretic.
Cilantro (Chinese Parsley)	Diuretic, calming and mildly sedative.
Dill	Flatulence, colic, milk flow promoting agent (glactagogue).
Garlic	Antimicrobial, used against high cholesterol, cancer and hypertension.
Marjoram	Indigestion, colic
Mint	Expectorant, colds, used as a local anesthetic, anti-spasmotic.
Onion	Asthma, colds, as an expectorant, against cancer.
Oregano	Anti-tussive (relieving or suppressing coughing), relief of rheumatism, vermifuge or antihelmintic (expels parasitic worms), diuretic, deodorizer.
Poppy Seed	Sedative, anti-spasmodic.

Rosemary	Anti-tumoral
Sage	Antiseptic, used for gastroenteritis and as a sedative.
Savory	Antispasmodic, sedative, vermifuge, diuretic.
Tarragon	Diuretic, vermifuge, emmenagogue.
Thyme	Expectorant, antiseptic.

(UCLA, 2002)

Essential Fatty Acids

Essential fatty acids are called essential because the body cannot manufacture certain fatty acids unless they are derived from foods containing them. The polyunsaturated omega 3 and omega 6 fatty acids the body needs for optimal health and preventing disease are derived from plant oils such as raw nuts, seeds, whole grains, edible flowers from herbs, fish and krill oils. Fatty acid supplements may include one or more of the above sources of fatty acids. The most common supplement sources of omega 3's and 6's are listed below.

Fish oils (eicosa-pentanoic acid or EPA)
Krill oil (derived from tiny crustaceans that are a food source for marine mammals and fish)
Flaxseed oil
Evening primrose oil
Borage oil

How the Body Uses Essential Fatty Acids

- Required by every type of cell in the body for maintaining the quality and function of cell membranes and inner organelle structures where the body's energy is produced, new proteins are synthesized, DNA gene sequencing is repaired, and cell replication and cell-differentiation is initiated.

- Required for the turnover and manufacture of every type of new cell, including the formation of hormones, immune cells, lubricating body fluids that protect joints, cartilage and connective tissues, and required to build, protect and maintain nerve and brain cell structures and functioning.

- Help provide sustained fuel efficiency throughout the day.

- Help nourish and maintain the strength and pliability of blood vessels and their cell membranes, including those of the heart and brain for maintaining safe blood pressure, particularly during exercise when extra pressure is exerted against blood vessel walls, and help maintain muscle tone and flexibility.

- Improve brain to nerve transmissions.

- Help prevent abnormal blood clotting.

- Are the precursors for the synthesis of the thousands of hormones that circulate and monitor the various body systems and regulate biochemical processes such as blood sugar, the immune system, pain nerve receptors, the fight or flight response, growth hormone, reproductive hormones, calcium regulation, blood pressure, heart rate, brain and nervous system functioning.

- Are essential in the maintenance of photo-receptor cells in the eyes and quality of skin.

- Are required for assisting in converting sun exposure on the skin to vitamin D3 (cholecalciferol) for stronger bones, immune function, hair growth, regulating body temperature, and forming protective, lubricating joint fluids.

- Help lower the amounts of lipids such as cholesterol and triglycerides in the blood.

- Essential for manufacturing the protective coating of the nerve cell's axon, the myelin sheath, which function is to help ensure correct impulse signaling between neurons throughout the nervous system that allows optimal brain functioning, quick reflex motor skills, and the activation and deactivation of billions of cell signaling processes throughout life.

Not all fats are created equal, for there are fats that are essential for optimal health, and there are processed or altered fats that result in damaging it. Fats that have been molecularly damaged or chemically or heat processed puts you at risk for several degenerative diseases, including cancer, heart disease, endocrine or glandular malfunctioning, diabetes, and various inflammatory conditions. Such health-damaging fats are known as trans fats.

Consuming trans fats interferes with cell functioning. Trans fats form free radicals that have been linked to cancer, heart disease, hormonal disruptions and glandular disorders, brain and nervous system disorders and other degenerative diseases. It is therefore critical for you to provide your body with fats that have their normal biocompatible molecular configurations intact, and avoid the altered fats with their unnatural molecular structures which the body perceives as foreign, invasive substances. Trans fats therefore should be absent from food choices, and definitely should not be present in a nutritional supplement.

All fatty acids contained in supplements therefore must be kept refrigerated in tightly closed containers to preserve the quality of their essential fatty acids. Both fatty acid supplements and whole foods containing essential fats must not be left exposed to air, for their highly vulnerable molecular structures make them prone to the undesirable and toxic oxidative process where volatile, free radical compounds damage cells that compose all body systems.

Flavonoids

Flavonoids used in nutritional supplements are derived from foods high in flavonoids, which the body converts to bioflavonoids. Like carotenoids, flavonoids are responsible for the brilliant colors of plants. Food flavonoids enhance vitamin absorption, and if a supplement you select contains flavonoids, it should also be accompanied with whole food sources of vitamin C.

Many whole food derived supplements do contain both vitamin C and flavonoids. Other supplements contain ascorbic acid, the synthetic form of vitamin C, along with what are listed as bioflavonoids. There are thousands of various types of flavonoids contained in plants, including their subclassifications. Below is a general breakdown of the most commonly known flavonoids and their whole food sources that commonly occur in nutritional supplements.

Anthocyanidins - Red, blue, purple berries, red and purple grapes, and red wine.

Flavanols - Catechins found in green and white teas, cocoa, grapes, berries, apples.

Flavanones - Citrus fruits and their juices such as grapefruits, lemons, oranges.

Flavonols (include quercetin, rutin, and hesperidin) - Yellow onions, scallions, kale, broccoli, apples, berries, teas.

Flavones - Parsley, thyme, celery, hot peppers.

Isoflavones - Soybeans, soy foods, legumes. (Linus, 2013)

Health benefits of flavonoids are:

- Strengthen capillaries and enhances their suppleness to prevent brittleness that can result in ruptures and breakages such as bruising or blood vessel damage.
- Prevent excessive inflammatory responses throughout the body and improve the behavior of the many different immune cells produced by the body.
- Effective against bacteria and viruses, including the HIV and HSV-1 herpes simplex viruses.
- Enhance the action of vitamin C.
- Function as antioxidants to help neutralize free radicals that scavenge healthy cells for electrons,

leaving cells damaged and vulnerable to mutagenic occurrences.
• Help increase the body's own glutathione levels, a powerful antioxidant that boosts the abilities of other antioxidants.
(Flavonoids 2013)

Individuals with a low intake of foods or supplements containing flavonoids may experience:

• Being prone to easy bruising
• Frequency of nose bleeds
• Excessive swelling from injuries
• Frequent viral or bacterial infections

Based on the scientific literature, studies indicate that even in amounts as high as 140 grams per day from nutritional supplements, or if are taken at 10% of total daily calorie intake, flavonoids do not appear to be toxic or put health at risk or produce undesirable side effects, including during pregnancy (Flavonoids 2013).

Fiber - Insoluble and Soluble

Many studies confirm the relationship between high fiber diets and many diseases such as heart disease, diabetes and cancer, and that plenty of fiber in the daily diet can prevent or treat constipation, hemorrhoids, and diverticulosis. Fiber supplement ingredients are derived from a wide variety of foods containing fiber, and can be purchased in capsule or tablet form, liquid form or powders that can be stirred or blended into a beverage or sprinkled on a meal.

There are two types of fiber: insoluble and water soluble, and most foods contain some of both.

Insoluble fiber:

- The undigestible fiber of plants. Enzymes produced in the human intestinal tract cannot digest this type of fiber; however, insoluble fiber serves to help mobilize bulk and remove waste from the colon.
- Metababolized by aerobic gut bacteria, which has many beneficial health effects, such as improving immune function, including overcoming anaerobic, pathogenic (illness or disease-causing) strains of bacteria. The colonies of beneficial bacteria or flora formed by ingesting insoluble fiber collectively act as a protective sub organ system within the colon or large intestine (O'Hara, 2006).
- Include foods that contain cellulose, hemicellulose and lignin.

Examples of foods containing insoluble fiber are barley, broccoli, brown rice, bulgur, cabbage, corn bran, carrots, celery, couscous, cucumbers, dark leafy vegetables, fruit, grapes, green beans, nuts, onions, raisins, root vegetable skins, seeds, tomatoes, wheat bran, whole grains and zucchini (Zelman).

Water soluble fiber:

- Attracts water into the intestine and forms a gel that slows down digestion and creates the feeling of being full.
- Helps decrease LDL cholesterol levels by preventing too much absorption of dietary cholesterol.
- Helps lower blood glucose

Examples of foods containing water soluble fiber are apples, beans, blueberries, carrots, celery, cucumbers, dried peas, flaxseeds, lentils, nuts, oat bran, oat cereal, oatmeal, oranges, pears, psyllium, and strawberries (Zelman).

Dietary guidelines for Americans are 25 grams for women under 50 and teenage girls, and 30-38 grams of dietary fiber for men under 50 and teenage boys. For good digestive health, the National Fiber Council recommends that children up to three years of age eat 19 grams of fiber per day, children aged four to eight, 25 grams, boys nine to thirteen, 31 grams, and girls nine to thirteen, 26 grams (Williams).

Digestive Aids

Contrary to popular belief, digestive problems such as "heart burn", flatulence or stomach pain are not necessarily due to the overproduction of stomach acids after a meal; in fact, it is often the under production of hydrochloric acid, bile acids, and pancreatic and liver enzymes required to complete the digestive process that creates various gastric upsets and sluggish intestinal mobilization. Diets lacking or low in raw foods results in deficiencies in metabolic, digestive and food enzymes needed to break down foods for proper assimilation and absorption. A digestive aid should therefore contain enzymes that help the body break down foods thoroughly so that nutrients can be absorbed more readily and utilized more completely.

Consuming digestive aids that contain calcium carbonate, or reaching for bicarbonate of soda to ease digestive upsets actually makes the problem worse. Such so-called digestive aids neutralize the essential hydrochloric acid normally excreted in the stomach. After swallowing, enzymes are needed to break down further the masticated food masses or bolluses in the stomach and small intestine. Various digestive enzymes are called into action to split the dense molecules of various proteins, fats and carbohydrates in various segments of the digestive tract, an essential preparation process required for further catabolizing simplified food substances down to their basic nutritional components in the intestines. As the food you eat is processed through the stomach and duodenum with the aid of pancreatic and liver enzymes, nutrients are then absorbed through the intestinal wall and absorbed into the blood stream for nutrient distribution throughout every body system.

Lacking adequate enzyme active, raw fresh foods in the daily diet interferes with complete and thorough digestion and nutrient absorption of cooked foods which enzymes are destroyed in heating and boiling temperatures, and reduces the body's ability to produce its own digestive acids and digestive enzymes. Enzymes are the catalysts of trillions of biological processes, or the sparks of life. For whatever challenge one might have in eating enough enzyme-active, raw foods, a digestive enzyme supplement dose taken before, with or after meals can help meet the body's vast metabolic enzyme requirements, aid digestion, prevent digestive upsets and improve nutrient absorption and utilization.

Types of Effective Digestive Aid Supplements

Prebiotics - A prebiotic is a nondigestible or partially digestible dietary fiber that nourishes the growth of healthy bacteria in the colon. The insoluble fibers of many fruits and vegetables are examples of foods that are prebiotics. Examples of foods high in prebiotic value are chicory root, wheat, onion, garlic, artichoke, oats, barley, legumes, kale, mustard and dandelion greens, dark green vegetables, and leeks. Prebiotic foods contain substances known as fructans that include native inulin, enzymatically hydrolized inulin or oligofructose or fructooligosaccharides that are listed on ingredient labels on supplements as FOS. Any of these ingredients found in your nutritional supplement selections are excellent.

Probiotics - Probiotics refers to the live microorganisms or beneficial aerobic bacteria that create a desirable, protective environment in the large intestine or colon. The most commonly used probiotics are lactobacillus and bifidobacteria. There are at least fifty types of lactobacillus and thirty types of bifidobacteria.

Lactobacillus has shown many benefits in studies for treating and preventing yeast and urinary tract infections, improving irritable bowel syndrome, restoring flora after antibiotic treatment, overcoming traveler's diarrhea infections, including from the pathogenic bacteria Clostridium difficile, and for restoring lactose intolerance, respiratory infections, and improving and alleviating various skin disorders such as canker sores, acne, eczema and fever blisters (Kovacs, 2013).

A group of researchers who studied the effects of the probiotic Lactobacillus reuteri on cancerous tumors concluded that future development of probiotic-based applications may prevent colorectal cancer and inflammatory bowel disease. Another study evaluated whether Lactobacillus acidophilus might improve immune functioning against human rotavirus infection that causes serious diarrhea in infants worldwide and a severe state of dehydration, and found that the probiotic promoted a better immune response in laboratory animals than when given a vaccine ("Two studies explore," 2008).

Lactobacilli that are in fermented foods such as live cultured yogurt, and as ingredients in nutritional supplements may include:

- L. acidophilus
- L. bulgaricus
- L. rhamnosus
- L. plantarium
- L. reuteri
- L. salivarius
- L. casei

(Kovacs, 2013)

Bifidobacteria consists of about 90% of healthy colon bacteria, and appears in the intestines of days old newborns and breastfed infants. In one four week study of 362 patients with irritable bowel syndrome, improvement in symptoms occurred with those who had been experiencing abdominal pain, bloating, constipation and gas. Bifidobacterium lactis reportedly lowered serum LDL cholesterol in type 2 diabetics and increased HDL cholesterol in women adults, as well as improved glucose tolerance in pregnant women.

The following are common bifidobacterium used in probiotic supplements:

- B. bifidum
- B. breve
- B. infantis
- B. lactis
- B. longum
- B. pseudolongum
- B. thermophilum

(Kovacs, 2013).

Probiotics are able to compete with illness causing or pathogenic microorganisms for sites within the colon. The probiotic beneficial bacteria establish themselves and cooperate with the body's immune response to modulate and reduce the effects of pathogenic microorganisms. Various clinical investigations conclude that probiotics may be useful for preventing and resolving a variety of health conditions such as:

- Allergies
- Cancers
- Cystic fibrosis
- Gastrointestinal infections
- Halitosis
- Inflammatory bowel disease
- Lactose intolerance
- Urogenital infections
- Reducing antibiotic side effects
- Reducing dental caries
- Periodontal disease

(Singh, 2013)

Tropical fruit enzymes - two enzymes commonly included in digestive aids and multi-nutrient supplements are bromelain from raw pineapple, and papain from raw papaya.

Bromelain

Bromelain is a complex of proteolytic or protein digesting enzymes from pineapples. It has been approved by the German Commission E for treatment of swelling and inflammation after surgery, including sinus, ear, nose and throat surgery, dental and foot surgery. Bromelain is also used to treat inflamed conditions from infection and physical injuries, including tendinitis, strains, bruising, and sprains, muscle and other minor injuries. It is also used to reduce trauma injuries.

Some studies show bromelain's nonsteroidal anti-inflammatory action, in combination with the flavonoid rutosid or rutin from buckwheat, and trypsin, an enzyme secreted by the pancreas as trypsinogen, worked as well as NSAIDs such as ibuprofen, naproxen and diclofenac and others, which indicated that bromelain may help ease pain for people with rheumatoid athritis.

There are some precautionary measures in the scientific literature when taking bromelain:

- May interact with some medications such as antibiotics, blood anticoagulants or antiplatelet drugs such as aspirin, warfarin or clopidogrel. It is also thought that bromelain may increase the effects of sedative medications, including antidepressants, anti-seizure, barbituates, benzodiazepines and alcohol. If you are taking *any* medication, consult with your trusted and knowledgeable health care provider.

- Bromelain is an effective protein digesting enzyme, and taking it longer than eight to ten days in a row is generally not advised.
- Those allergic to pineapples, celery, carrots, fennel, papain, pollen or wheat also may be allergic to bromelain.
- If one experiences mild nausea, diarrhea, vomiting or excessive menstrual bleeding, notify your health care provider and cease taking bromelain.
- Avoid bromelain if you have a bleeding disorder, high blood pressure, or disease of the kidney or liver.
- Do not take bromelain two weeks prior to surgery.
- Caution should also be considered if you are taking catnip, kava and valerian herbs while taking bromelain.

(University of Maryland Medical Center, 2013)

Papain

Historically, papain has been used for allergies, sports injuries and other causes of physical trauma. A protease enzyme, studies show that papain helps the body heal athletes' minor injuries more rapidly compared to placebos, and cuts recovery time in half. Papain has also been shown to alleviate allergies linked to leaky gut syndrome, insufficient stomach acid production, and gluten intolerance. Papain has also been reported as having anti-inflammatory and analgesic properties in sinus pain, headache and toothaches (Amri, 2012).

As with other proteolytic enzymes, the same precautions should be considered as those outlined in the Bromelain section above.

Raw apple cider vinegar - To receive the full benefit of the cider vinegar, choose the raw, enzyme-active product. It can be purchased in liquid form, where you can add a small amount to water, green drinks, or use as a salad dressing. Raw cider vinegar can also be purchased in tablet form.

Raw apple cider vinegar has been used for centuries for all manner of ailments: as a digestive aid, for easing pain, sinus infections, chronic fatigue, weight loss, improving the body's acid-alkaline pH balance, sore throats, kidney stones, nausea, asthma, insect bites, warts, easing heartburn, as a mouthwash diluted with water, a teeth whitener, and more.

In one study, apple cider vinegar showed promise for use in diabetic therapy where it helped reduce insulin resistance, which occurs when muscle, fat and liver cells do not respond properly to insulin (Johnston, 2013). In another clinical trial with type 1 diabetic patients, it was concluded that apple cider vinegar could help reduce hyperglycemia (Panayota, 2010). Secreted by the pancreas, insulin normally assists in the efficient uptake of glucose into the cells, but as the continuous presence of too much refined sugar and refined starch calls upon the pancreas to secrete ever higher amounts of insulin, sugar uptake is eventually impaired when the beta cells in the pancreas cannot keep up with the sugar load. A chronic excess glucose build up in the bloodstream leads to prediabetes, then type 2 diabetes. Excess dietary refined sugars and other carbohydrates lead to obesity and other associated disease risks (Insulin, 2013).

Digestive Enzymes - Some multi-nutrient vitamin-mineral supplements in tablet or powder form may consist of any combination of probiotics, prebiotics, tropical fruit enzymes and cider vinegar. Multi-nutrient supplements also usually contain metabolic enzymes normally found in typical digestive enzyme tablets, which are amylase, protease, and lipase. The body should be able to manufacture these food digesting enzymes on its own but may not produce sufficient amounts if the diet is deficient in enough fresh, raw foods. The amylase, protease and lipase enzymes digest carbohydrates, proteins and fats, respectively.

- Amylase - breaks down complex carbohydrates or starches to the most simple sugar units, glucose.
- Protease - breaks down protein foods such as meats, poultry, fish and dairy down to the basic components of life, amino acids.
- Lipase - breaks down dietary fats and oils to the fundamental units of fatty acids.

A digestive aid containing the above metabolic enzymes can provide a significant difference in how you feel after ingesting a heavy or high calorie meal, or if you just want to ensure you are utilizing nutrients in your food optimally.

Digestive aids or multi-nutrient supplements that include amylase, protease, lipase , fruit enyzmes, raw apple cider vinegar, probiotics and prebiotics in their formulas are great choices for enhancing your body's digestion, nutrient absorption capacity and metabolic activities. However, dietary enzymes and flavonoids derived from fresh foods remains important for ensuring that the body is able to produce its own metabolic and digestive enzymes too.

Spices

Derived from the word "species" back in the Middle Ages, spices include groups of fragrant and pungent, exotic food substances that have been used for flavorings and effective medicines through the ages. Spices have also been used as a valuable currency that has defined wealthy economies in Europe and Asia since time immemorial, and showcased the amount of wealth and power possessed by countries and individuals.

The use and characterization that defines the general term, "spice" may include an exotic or tropical part of an herbal plant that provides color, distinctive stimulating odor or aromatic fragrance. This can include typical culinary herbs such as mint, basil, thyme, rosemary, sage, fennel, garlic, onion and chives; pungents such as mustard, horseradish, peppers, peppercorns, coriander and turmeric; and the distinctive tastes of chocolate, coffee, teas, wine and olive or other oils, all of which provide unique scents and aromas to foods and beverages. Spicy aromatic scents such as cardamom, ginger, cloves, nutmeg, allspice, cinnamon, cassia, myrrh, saffron, anise and licorice are used in condiments, sweets, cordials, liqueurs, cosmetics, medications and fragrances.

Any one or more of the above spices may be found in nutritional supplements and alternative medicines administered by medical practitioners throughout the world outside of Western medicine. Spices have been used for thousands of years as flavor enhancements to improve the taste of foods, and have been used as preservatives against food spoilage and preventing illness caused by pathogenic or illness-causing organisms such as viruses, bacteria, parasites or fungi, or used as antidotes for poisons or venoms.

Spices have been potent therapeutic foods and medicinals for many types of ailments dating back to pre-biblical times for the Greeks, Romans, medieval Europeans, Africans, Asians and Middle Easterners. Additionally, many exotic spices have been noted for their aphrodisiac effects. Today, spices are used in all medical systems throughout the world. In addition to their antimicrobial, anticatarrhal or nasal mucous dissipating attributes and gastrointestinal antithelmintic and other beneficial properties, spices are also effective as pest repellents, although pungent spices are not always unattractive to birds or rodents.

In the following tables below are listed the nutritional values of the more commonly used spices, and that are used in medical systems outside of Western medicine. Spices are used in various cultural, naturopathic medicinal formulations and also found in many nutritional supplements.

Phytonutrients in Spices

Over millions of years, plants that fall into the defined category of spices have acquired a diverse amount of phytochemicals or phytonutrients, which serve to repel pathogenic, or illness or disease causing organisms. The phytonutrients in spices inhibit the invasion of pathogenic bacteria, viruses, fungi and parasitic worms and have high antioxidant and enzyme activity. Studies show that there are certain bacterial infections associated with certain cancer risks, and viruses are now known to be the second highest cause of cancer in humans.

Spices possess properties shown to inhibit mutagenesis or abnormal cell replication cycles, preventing damage to DNA that leads to cancerous conditions. Spices inhibit the proliferation and progression of cancer cell cycle processes and can induce apoptosis, or cancer cell self-destruction, by improving the mechanisms that contribute to cancer, which are lowered immune function, inflammation, and imbalanced hormone metabolism.

In general, phytochemicals function to attract beneficial organisms such as oxygen loving aerobic bacteria or probiotic organisms, and repel harmful anaerobic organisms that thrive in low oxygen environments. The antioxidant activity in spices neutralize free radicals that would otherwise inflict DNA damage. Spices have also been analyzed for their anti-inflammatory capacity (Lampe, 2003).

There are literally thousands of phytochemicals that are currently being studied. Many of the commonly used spice plants contain many of the same phytonutrients, while they also contain some of their own unique phytochemicals. The list below will familiarize you with some common phytochemicals found in spices and other foods used in nutritional supplements.

- **Alkaloids** - bitter amines: capsaicin, caffeine, theobromine, theophylline.
- **Coumarins** - aromatic lactones: hydroxycoumarins, furanocoumarins, pyranocoumarins, benzopyrones.
- **Flavonoids** - plant pigments: luteolin, myricetin, proanthocyanidins, catechins, epicatechins, quercetin, rutin.
- **Essential oils** - coumarins, limonene, eugenol, beta-caryophyllene, terpenine, sesquiterpene.
- **Glycosides** - sugar esters, derivatives from carbohydrates: allinin, saponins, anthocyanins.
- **Phenols** - volatile oils or aromatic compounds: phenolic acids, phenolic diterpenes, flavonoids, stilbenoids, curcumin.
- **Phenylpropanoids** - eugenol, phenolic acids, esters, glycosylated derivatives of primary PPPs, flavonoids, isoflavonoids, stilbenes, coumarins, curcuminoids, lignans.
- **Resins** - terpene oxidants, resin acids.
- **Saponins** - soapy hemolysants: glycyrrhizin.
- **Sterols** - plant steroidal chemicals: hundreds of precursors required for production of the body's thousands of regulating hormones.
- **Tannins** - polyphenolics: catechins, proanthocyanidins.
- **Terpenes** - isoprene derivatives: zingiberene, monoturpines, sesquiterpenes, diterpenes.

(Medicinal Plants, 2011), (UCLA, 2002), (Phytochemicals, n.d.), (Shan, 2005), (Tacouri, 2013)

Spices Categorized According to Traditional Uses by Medical Systems Outside of Western Medicine

Hot, Pungent, Exotic	
Allspice	Used against vomiting and nausea (anti-emetic), has a strong laxative effect (purgative).
Capsicum (peppers)	Anti-inflammatory, pain relief (analgesic), expectorant.
Cassia	Antiseptic, used to counter diarrhea.
Cinnamon	(See Cassia)
Clove	Used as a topical anesthetic, for indigestion, soothing a person's irritable disposition.
Coriander	Used against spasms, a diuretic, an anti-inflammatory agent.
Cumin	Anti-microbial, expels parasitic worms (vermifuge), a diuretic.
Curry leaves	Used to calm vomiting and nausea.
Ginger	Used for colds, sore throats, alleviate nausea, against vomiting, and for rheumatic pain relief.
Mace	Body tissues and skin tightening effect (astringent).
Nutmeg	(See Mace)
Peppercorns	Expectorant, destroys pathogenic (illness causing) organisms.
Saffron	Used to sooth rheumatism, relief of nerve pain (neuralgia).
Turmeric	Used for arthritic pain, is a potent antioxidant, used against cancer.
Wasabi	Effective expectorant, used to alleviate sinusitis.

(UCLA, 2002)

Hot, Pungent, Non-Exotic	
Horseradish	Antimicrobial, used as an expectorant and purgative (laxative effect).
Mustard	Anti-inflammatory agent, purgative, can be used as an emetic (encourage vomiting).
Paprika	Used as a colorant, is an anti-inflammatory, a good natural source of Vitamin C (ascorbic acid).

(UCLA, 2002)

Warm, Fragrant, Exotic	
Aniseed	Used as an anti-spasmodic, an expectorant, and is a mild sedative.
Bergamot	Has antiseptic properties, an anti-spasmodic, mild sedative.
Caraway	Diuretic, anti-spasmodic, aids in production of mothers milk (galactagogue)
Cardamom	Has antiseptic properties.
Carob	Used as an astringent, purgative, diuretic.
Chocolate	Mild sedative effects, diuretic.
Coffee	Stimulant, diuretic, dilates bronchial tubes.
Kola nut	Used to calm or prevent vomiting, an astringent.
Fennel	Anti-spasmodic, diuretic.
Fenugreek	Effective for controlling blood sugar, helps maintain healthy blood cholesterol levels.
Juniper	Antiseptic, used to ease rheumatism, diuretic, used to induce perspiration (sudorific).
Lemon Grass	Used for fever, repels insects.

Licorice	Used for coughs (antitussive), spasms, and peptic ulcer.
Nigella	Used to expel parasites, used as a laxative (purgative), and is a diuretic.
Sesame seed	Used to promote mother's milk production, a diuretic, used to soothe or soften as in soothing and coating an irritated throat during a cold.
Star anise	Has antiseptic and anti-rheumatic properties.
Tea	Anti-oxidant.
Vanilla	Helps reduce fever (febrifuge or antipyretic) and spasms.

(UCLA, 2002)

6 The "Other Ingredients" on Your Supplement Label - What To Avoid

Toxic, Potentially Toxic or Allergenic Ingredients in Nutritional Supplements

The following are used as fillers or excipients that bind tablets together:

- Corn starch, particularly from GMO corn
- Microcrystalline cellulose
- Silicon dioxide
- Titanium dioxide
- Sodium starch glycolate
- Lactose
- Talc
- Sucrose
- Hydroxy propyl methylcellulose
- Croscamellose
- Calcium phosphate
- Ethyl cellulose
- Shellac

- Parafin

The chemicals listed below are sometimes used in cheap brands. These chemicals enter the circulatory system upon skin contact or oral ingestion. They end up stored in the liver, heart, kidneys and muscles for several years and can cause skin rashes, dandruff, hair loss, eye irritations and allergic reactions.

- Propylene glycol - present in antifreeze, windshield washer, brake and hydraulic fluids. Used in cosmetics, deodorants, shampoos and body lotions. Is documented as causing kidney and liver damage.
- Sodium laurel sulfate and sodium laureth sulfate - used as detergent foaming agent, is found in garage floor cleaners, car wash soap and engine degreasers. Found in shampoo and cosmetics. Interact with other ingredients in many consumer products to form carcinogenic nitrates and dioxins.

Other hazardous ingredients:

- BHT
- BHA
- Polysorbate 80
- Tartrazine
- Red dye 33 and 40
- Hydrogenated or fractionated oils
- Ethyl cellulose
- Fractionated cornstarch

- GMO ingredients from genetically altered foods (not organically grown): corn, sugar beets, alfalfa, zucchini, golden rice, soy, yeast, cassava, banana, potatoes, corn, tomatoes, cottonseed, corn, canola and soy oil, and cows, pigs and chickens are fed

GMO corn.

Nontoxic and Naturally Derived Ingredients

- Stearic acid - a natural fatty acid made by humans and animals that is converted in the body to oleic acid, a fatty acid necessary for good health.
- Magnesium stearate - used as an excipient to prevent supplement ingredients from sticking or clumping to the manufacturing equipment.

In the mass production of chemicals and drugs, some of those substances do not interact well with magnesium stearate merely due to the nature of their molecular structure. However, the human body's biochemical interactions utilize magnesium stearate completely differently than the nonbiological chemical reactions of synthetic substances that occur in a laboratory. An accumulation of years of scientific data points to the fact that magnesium stearate, derived from combining calcium or magnesium with stearic acid, which is derived from vegetable oils and made by the body, does not pose any health threat.

Because a study showing that when human immune cells were exposed to impossibly high concentrations of stearic acid (which is completely different from magnesium stearate) in the effort to prevent rejection of transplanted organs, researchers found that stearic acid suppressed the immune function of those T cells. In this study, there were no oral intakes of magnesium stearate. Because of this study, there have been reports in the media that magnesium stearate is hazardous to health. However, since it is a natural substance the body comfortably and easily converts to a natural fatty acid, oleic acid, it has not been found to pose any health threat (Dever, 2013).

- Gelatin - a type of protein derived by the partial hydrolysis of collagen from the skin, bones and connective tissue of animals such as cattle, chicken, fish and pigs. It is used in foods and drugs as a thickening agent such as for salad dressings, and as a suspension medium such as jello, jelly or other desserts.

Gelatin is also derived from the hemi-cellulose of plants to provide alternative choices for those with allergies to certain animal products, and for vegetarians. When combined with water and then dried in the manufacturing process, gelatin can be shaped into capsules for drugs and nutritional supplements.

Non-Absorbable Minerals

- Egg shell, oyster shell calcium
- Elemental minerals (not listed on the product label as anything other than the mineral itself)
- Mineral oxides

Disruptive to Digestion

- Calcium carbonate - reduces essential hydrochloric acid required for proper digestion.
- Various grades of tablet coatings of animal origin.
- Hydrogenated oils listed as "Other Ingredients" on a product label.
- Elemental minerals.

- Synthetic vitamins.

Synthetic Versions of Vitamins

- Synthetic vitamin A - retinyl acetate, retinol acetate, vitamin A acetate, vitamin A palmitate, retinyl palmitate, 13-cis-retinoic acid and retinoids. Ingestion of excess doses of vitamin A may produce such symptoms as abdominal pain, anemia, liver disease, eczema, edema, hair loss, headache, lethargy, respiratory/lung infection and vomiting.

- Synthetic B complex vitamins made from petro chemicals:
  Synthetic Thiamine (Vitamin B1) - Thiamine mononitrate, thiamine hydrochloride
  Synthetic Riboflavin (Vitamin B2) - Riboflavin pantothenic acid, calcium D-pantothenate
  Synthetic Pyridoxine (Vitamin B6) - Pyridoxine hydrochloride
  Synthetic Cobalamin (PABA or para-aminobenzoic acid) - Aminobenzoic acid
  Synthetic Folic Acid - Pteroylglutamic acid
  Synthetic Choline - Choline chloride, choline bitartrate
  Synthetic Biotin - d-Biotin

  Niacin (Vitamin B3) - nicotinic acid and niacinamide make up vitamin B3, and is derived naturally from the essential amino acid tryptophan found in animal protein foods. Along with the other B vitamins, B3 is found in animal-derived proteins and in green vegetables, cereal grains and yeast. Isolated niacinamide is used in most B complex nutritional supplements as the vitamin B3 component.

- Synthetic vitamin C - ascorbic acid. Can be found in combination with naturally occurring forms of vitamin C such as from amla berries, ascerola cherries, rose hips, or peppers. Manufacturers use the synthetic version of vitamin C to raise the number of milligrams of each tablet, or serving size in the case of the powdered form. However, absorbability and usability is the real concern when choosing a vitamin C supplement, and not necessarily the alleged potency.

- Synthetic vitamin D - irradiated ergosteral, calciferol, calcitriol, doxercalciferol and calcipotriene.

   Vitamin D poisoning is rare; however, per the Organic Consumers Association, "Toxicity can occur under certain medical conditions such as primary hyperparathyroidism, tuberculosis and lymphoma." When produced by the body itself from exposure to UV sunlight, there is no risk of Vitamin D toxicity.

- Synthetic vitamin E - dl-alpha tocopherol, dl-alpha tocopherol acetate or succinate.

   According to the Organic Consumers Association, excess doses of synthetic vitamin E "may result in allergic reaction, breathing impairments, swelling of the tongue, fatigue, headache, nausea, blurred vision, excessive bleeding (anticoagulation due to inhibition of vitamin K), increased oxidative stress, increased hypertension, decreased life span."

- Synthetic vitamin K (menadione) - The Organic Consumers Association says "supplementation with a synthetic form of vitamin K Menadione has been associated with liver damage. Some reports indicate a significant association between high intramuscular levels of vitamin K and cancer." (Hofmekler, 2009)

Over 95% of vitamin supplements available today are in the synthetic category. Some vitamins are 100% synthesized while some are combinations of synthetic and naturally-occurring vitamins from foods and botanicals, including yeasts and algae. Comparatively few vitamin supplements currently on the market are derived from such whole food sources. When manufacturers label their supplements as "natural", the contents may not all be naturally derived from whole foods sources.

As long as there are some naturally derived substances in their supplement formulations, manufacturers can make label claims that their product is from natural sources. This misleading labeling is a source of confusion and is deceitful to the unwary consumer. If a label does not say "naturally occurring" and does not list the food source from which it was derived, chances are the supplement may contain synthetic vitamins or synthetic chemicals.

More consumers need to get involved in encouraging truth in labeling mandates, following such organizations' activities such as the Naturally Occurring Standards Group (NOSG), the Hippocrates Health Institute, Healthful Communications, Inc., and the Organic Consumers Association. For twenty years, the

Hippocrates Institute has examined blood samples of thousands of people who had been taking synthetic vitamins. Researchers found that the body perceives a synthetic substance as a foreign invader and responds by mobilizing its white blood cells or leukocytes to attack what it perceives to be a health threat. While the immune system is attempting to rid itself of the foreign substances, other immune system functioning is compromised, with less capacity for destroying viruses, bacteria, parasites or spirochetes, or effectively preventing mutagenic cells from turning into cancer. Taking synthetic forms of vitamins, therefore, leave one more vulnerable to the disease process (Clement, 2006).

The differences between the molecular structures of synthetic vitamins versus those extracted from whole food is like looking at a schematic drawing of a house plan and the physical house itself. The combinations of carbon, hydrogen and oxygen atoms may look similar when depicted in diagrams, but the multi-dimensional configuration and full spectrum matrix of vitamins derived from whole foods are readily absorbed and utilized. With a synthetic vitamin, the body must search the entire system in the effort to complete the missing factors that would be present in a natural vitamin complex. The body must initiate biochemical actions in the effort to prevent damage, using up more of the body's resources and reserves.

Vitamins are optimally utilized when the whole vitamin complex is present in its entirety as it exists in a whole food. If only an extracted component of the vitamin complex is used, such as a single B vitamin for example, the body cannot absorb more than 50% of the extract, and even less is utilized to health advantage when ingesting synthetic vitamins. It is best therefore to select supplements containing whole foods when choosing them for their vitamin content.

The human body simply cannot "digest" synthetic chemicals. Instead, synthetic vitamins may create inflammatory conditions throughout since they are not readily absorbable. Even if they are allowed past the cell membrane into the manufacturing, disassembling and repurposing facilities inside the cells, rather than facilitating, and due to many missing components of those molecular structures, synthetic vitamins can interfere with the process of generating essential new proteins, sugars and fatty acids needed to build new tissues, fluids and structures in any body system. Synthetics may impair the maintenance and performance of various body systems, such as the digestive, urinary, respiratory, lymph, cardiovascular, skeletal, muscular, glandular, immune and brain and nervous systems.

As you know, you are what you eat, what you digest, and ultimately, what you absorb, and that fresh, whole foods contain the food enzymes that help with digestion and the absorption of vitamins and minerals, and to manufacture metabolic enzymes , hormones, tissues, structures and all new body proteins. What you eat determines how well your body can maintain optimal conditions throughout your entire system. However, there is one more aspect or dimension to health vibrancy that is missed in typical nutritional literature and by nutritional advisors. With cutting edge scientific research in emerging new fields of biophysics known as biophotonics and bioenergy, a new way of examining the energy-transferring value of foods is being revealed.

Research showing the bioenergy fields and energy frequencies of naturally derived versus synthetic vitamins shows why the body cannot absorb and utilize their synthetic versions.

Researchers have found that by passing a beam of polarized light through a natural vitamin and its so-called chemically identical, synthetic version, the great differences between their bioavailability can be revealed. When passed through a natural vitamin, the beam of light bends to the right because of the direction of its molecular positioning showing its rotation. When passed through a synthetic vitamin, half the beam of light bends to the right, and the other half is bent to the left, rendering it non-absorbable and unable to pass through the highly sensitive cell surface receptor sites on the outer plasma cell membrane, which are programmed to only accept specific and proper matching molecular blueprints.

Therefore, naturally derived, full spectrum vitamins are essential for full absorbability and usability at the micro cell level, where true health is determined. Proper molecular configurations of naturally derived, whole vitamin complexes allow the body to manufacture fully functioning immune cells that help control inflammatory conditions when it detects foreign invasive particles or pathogenic organisms. A properly functioning immune system can correctly determine the level of threat to the system, properly respond to a particular threat, and thus be better able to eliminate it efficiently and effectively.

It must be noted that it is important to be aware that the term "natural" is a non-regulated term used by the food, supplement and natural products industries liberally and which product descriptions are not necessarily based on nature. The phrase "naturally derived" does not always indicate that a product's vitamin content includes a whole food vitamin complex, or that a whole botanical is present in any formulation. Many supplements list the name of the botanical on the label; however, a supplement may only contain a certain extract or extracted phytochemical or nutrient, as opposed to the whole plant containing its entire spectrum of synergistic nutrients and biochemicals.

Also be aware that the Food and Drug Administration's (FDA) standards of Recommended Daily Allowances (RDA) are now referred to as Daily Values (DV's) and Recommended Daily Intakes (RDI's) for vitamins, and are based on nutrient values of synthetic versions (NOSG). As you compare potencies on labels between the vitamin values of a whole food nutrient supplement with a synthetic supplement, know that higher potencies aren't always an indication of absorbability. If whole food vitamin complexes are present in the supplement, your absorbability rate is likely 100%. Multi-whole food ingredients concentrated in a supplement that offers pansystemic, deep cell absorption and utilization value is therefore a wiser choice than a high potency synthetic version with little use and possible systemic aggravation.

A new consumer standard in referencing vitamins and other nutrient values, called the Naturally Occurring Standard (NOS), is being proposed, where manufacturers can display on nutritional supplement labeling and food panel ingredient lists naturally-occurring nutrients. This would help buyers of such goods select foods and supplements with higher whole food value and therefore a more complete range of nutrients. The greater the disclosure on food and supplement labeling, the more product buyers as a whole can raise the levels of nutritional health for themselves and their families (Clement, 2006).

Additives or "Other Ingredients" Listed on Product Labels

Nutritional supplement tablets are coated with various grades of shellac or vegetable glaze. Tablets may contain many types of tablet binders and fillers, which are also used for topping off gelatin capsules. Many supplements contain coloring agents--all of which can be potentially allergenic, aggravate tissues and affect nutrient absorption. If you select supplements with the least amount of additives in the "Other Ingredients" list on the product's label, the higher are the chances of you being able to absorb and utilize its nutrients. Depending on what "Other Ingredients" in a supplement consist of, it can make the difference between 90% or more of its absorbability versus an absorbability rate of 25% or lower. The only advantage of using potentially allergenic substances in supplements is to expedite the manufacturing process, and not necessarily to serve in the best interest of the health conscious consumer (Schmid, 2002).

Artificial Colorings

Food colorings are found in beverages, candy, cereals, sweets and baked goods.

- **Blue 1** - Studies indicate possible cancer risk, affects neurons, causes occasional allergic reactions.

- **Blue 2** - Evidence shows it may cause brain cancer in male rats.

- **Citrus Red 2** - Artificial coloring in some Florida oranges. Rarely used and therefore indicates small risk. Toxic to rodents and caused bladder tumors.

- **Green 3** - Hints of tumors in bladder and reproductive organs in male rats, possibly carcinogenic.

- **Orange B** - High doses harmful to liver and bile duct.

- **Red 3** - Convincing evidence that causes thyroid tumors in rats.

- **Red 40** - Can cause allergy-like reactions and may trigger hyperactivity in children.

- **Yellow 5** - Causes allergy-like hypersensitivity reactions, triggers hyperactivity in children. May be contaminated with carcinogens benzidine and 4-aminbiphenyl or other chemicals that cause the body to convert them to those substances.

- **Yellow 6** - Causes tumors of the adrenal gland and kidney. Contains contaminant carcinogens benzidine and 4-aminbiphenyl or other chemicals that cause the body to convert them to those substances. May cause hypersensitivity reactions (Kobylewski, 2010).

Sweeteners

- **Aspartame (Equal, NutraSweet)** - Artificial sweetener. There has been much controversy for decades over whether aspartame causes cancer or neurological problems such as dizziness or hallucinations. In 2007 studies showed that rats given aspartame throughout their lifespan developed lymphomas, leukemias, kidney tumors, lung cancer, liver and mammary gland cancer.

- **High fructose corn syrup -** (as well as other sugars) has been linked to obesity, heart disease, diabetes, tooth decay, gout (arthritis), high blood pressure, high blood sugar and triglycerides, lowers good cholesterol. Corn undergoes a long process to become high fructose corn syrup. It is highly refined and linked to obesity, diabetes, heart disease and cancer. It limits the body's ability to detect when it is full, causes mineral imbalances, is converted to fat more so than other sugars, increases uric acid production that can cause inflammation and joint pain. Corn syrup also may contain low levels of the dangerous element, mercury.

  HFCS is made from genetically modified corn where neonicotinoid pesticides are spliced into the DNA of corn to make them resistant to insects. Colony Collapse Disorder (CCD) has destroyed millions of bee colonies since the introduction of neonicotinoid pesticides to crops due to how it destroys their nervous systems (Hance, 2012). Pesticides are also linked to serious environmental devastation, and have affected millions of essential pollinators such as honey bees, bumble bees and butterflies. Without pollinator insects, over 50% of the world's foods would be destroyed since pollination is essential to a plant or tree's food production (Tapparo, 2012).

Pesticides are linked to prostate, ovarian, melanoma or other skin cancers, brain and nervous system damage and birth defects. Pesticides are known hormone disruptors, accumulate in the body's tissues and are passed on to newborns ("Cancer").

HFCS is used in baked goods, candy bars, breakfast cereals, and can be in any other processed food product or beverage.Public health departments in major and other cities across the U.S. have supported a proposal to reduce sugars in soft drinks and other products. The average American consumes about 78 lbs of sugar additives per year.

Sugar Additives Consumed by Americans Per Year

6 lbs per month
3 ounces or 9 tbsps per day
36 lbs of cane or beet sugar* or (sucrose)
*beet sugar is also genetically modified
29 lbs of high fructose corn syrup
9 lbs corn sugar
1 lb honey

The Center for Science in the Public Interest urges the FDA to determine a safe level of sugar to try to get Americans to reduce their dangerously high sugar intake, particularly if GMOs are present. It would be wise to leave highly refined sweeteners, including GMO HFCS, out of any nutritional protocol, and they certainly do not have any value in any nutritional supplement.

- **Saccharin (Sweet 'N Low)** - Artificial sweetener. Used as a sugar substitute and is 350 times sweeter than sugar. Used as a tabletop sweetener.

  National Cancer Institute found that saccharin can cause cancer of the urinary bladder.

  Other studies showed that it can cause cancer of the female reproductive organs, skin, blood vessels and other organs.

  Other studies show it increases the potent carcinogenic activity of other chemical carcinogens.

  In 1977, the FDA announced that saccharin should be banned because of studies showing it caused cancer in animals, but Congress intervened and only required label warnings.

  In 1997, the diet-food industry pressured the U.S. and Canada and the World Health Organization to exclude saccharin from cancer-causing chemicals list, knowing the results of scientific studies.

  In 2000, saccharin was removed from the list of cancer-causing chemicals by the U.S. Department of Health and Human Services, and a law was passed by Congress to remove the cancer warning notice on labels.

- **Sucralose (Splenda)** - Artificial sweetener. Added

to baked goods, ice cream, soft drinks, and used as a tabletop sweetener.

Approved in the U.S. in 1998.

The Center for Science in the Public Interest states sucralose is safer than other artificial sweeteners.

Unlike aspartame, it does not break down at high oven temperatures so can be used for baking.

Studies attempting to show any health hazards in consuming aspartame are varied:

- One animal study indicated it might shrink the thymus gland, which function is essential for the immune system, but another study did not find this problem.
- Studies attempting to show sucralose could cause cancer did not find such results or any other problems.
- A 2002 animal study showed huge doses damaged DNA in mice, but other genetic studies found no problems.
- A 2012 study discovered that sucralose and saccharin may reduce gut bacteria and digestive enzymes, and therefore contribute to irritable bowel disease (IBD) with severe cramping and pain, ongoing diarrhea and rectal bleeding.

Note: Artificial sweeteners are more common in processed foods now , so read ingredient lists on product labels if you wish to avoid them.

Other Common Food Additives

• **Hydrogenated oils (Trans fats)**

Margarine - used in processed oil products such as mayonnaise and salad dressings, baked goods, icing, microwave popcorn. Margarine and shortening are formed when a vegetable oil is converted into a solid by a manufacturing process using a chemical reaction with hydrogen known as hydrogenation. This process forms trans fats, which damage healthy cells.

Hydrogenated oils and shortening are associated with heart disease, cancer and other serious conditions. In 2004, the U.S. Food and Drug Administration (FDA) announced that gram for gram, trans fats are harmful. The Institute of Medicine advises that people consume less than 2 grams a day or 7/100 of an ounce.

The Harvard School of Public Health estimates that 50,000 premature deaths from heart attack per year has been caused by trans fat and said that "This makes partially hydrogenated oil one of the most harmful ingredients in the food supply.". As of 2006, nutrition labels have been required to list the amount of trans fats per serving. Since 2000 and as of 2007, consumption of trans fats have been reduced by 50%. The cities of New York, Philadelphia and Boston have set limits on the amount of trans fats in restaurant foods.

- **Sodium Benzoate** - A study in the UK showed hyperactivity and attention deficit in 4 year old children given sodium benzoate, and altered their behavior. Behavior improved during the withdrawal phase after receiving drinks containing 20 mg of artificial coloring and 45 mg of sodium benzoate daily, and there was an increase in hyperactive behavior during the active period compared to the placebo group.In the early 1990's drink manufacturers were requested to fix this problem in their ingredients, but didn't get around to it for another ten years until after there were many lawsuits. Sodium benzoate, when combined with ascorbic acid and added heat forms benzene, a human carcinogen.

- **Sodium Nitrite,** - A preservative used against illness causing bacteria such as clostridium botulinum contamination, retains meat coloring (keeps meat from looking gray) and used as a flavoring for bacon, corned beef, ham, frankfurters and lunch meats.

- **Sodium Nitrate** - Used to dry and cure meat and breaks down to nitrite in the body.

  It has been found that both nitrite and nitrate may lead to forming cancer-causing nitrosamines in the body, especially in fried bacon, so ascorbic acid or erthorbic acid is added to it to reduce the amount of nitrosamines produced.

  Freezing and refrigeration prevents the botulinum and other illness causing bacteria from increasing, but not for as long.

The U.S. Department of Agriculture developed a safe method to prevent botulism poisoning using lactic-acid producing bacteria (lactic acid is produced by the body).

- **BHA -** Used in cereals, chewing gum, potato chips, vegetable oil.

  Retards rancidity in fats, oils and foods and products containing oils.

  Some studies consider it safe, while other studies show it causes cancer in rats, mice and hamsters in their forestomachs, which humans do not have. However, the studies are considered valid because if a chemical causes cancer in one organ in three different species, it may be carcinogenic in humans.

  The U.S. Food and Drug Administration permits BHA to be used in foods as a "reasonably anticipated to be a human carcinogen" additive.

- **BHT -** Used in cereals, chewing gum, potato chips, oils.

  Retards rancidity in oils.

  Animal studies showed either an increased or decreased risk of cancer.

  BHT is not necessary and easily replaced by safe additives.

- **Brominated vegetable oil (BVO)** - Used as an emulsifier in citrus-flavored drinks to keep flavorings from separating and floating to the top.

PepsiCo decided to stop using brominated vegetable oil in Gatorade, also referred to as BVO, as the result of consumer pressure.

In January, 2013, Gatorade decided to reformulate the beverage thanks to a petition started by a fifteen year old girl that ended up with over 200,000 signatures that got the Gatorade corporation's attention.

In two documented cases, those who drank BVO-laced beverages heavily suffered from bromide intoxication, with symptoms of memory loss and neurological problems.

Scientists say bromide accumulates in human tissue: the body's fat deposits, brain tissue, cartilage, liver, spinal fluids, mother's milk.

Two scientific studies found that when rodents nursing their young were fed brominated olive oil or BVO, their normal development was affected, and concern was raised that it may have the same effect on human children.

Brominated chemicals are used widely in tv sets and other electronics, and as flame retardants for foam furniture.

Brominated chemicals are linked to hormone disruptions and affect neurodevelopment. The U.S. Food and Drug Administration allowed its use in soft drinks in 1977, but is banned from European and Japanese soft drinks (Gilbert, 2013).

Note: Do not hesitate to request full disclosure of all ingredients and manufacturing processes from a manufacturer. The more they are willing to disclose to you about their product, the better you can trust it. Experience has shown that if a company is evasive or non-communicative, it is likely to be coincidental that they will not want to discuss their product ingredients, and those ingredients may very well be questionable.

7 Final Do's and Don'ts for Selecting Supplements

Don'ts:

Never select a supplement based on price. Always base your decision on nutrient density and absorbability, from naturally derived ingredients.

Never choose a supplement based on supposing a high end name brand contains the best ingredients. Corporate conglomerates regularly buy out smaller supplement companies and their emphasis is not often about quality, but quantity and high profit margins.

Avoid supplements containing GMOs. See Chapter Two for more information about genetically modified organisms.

Try to avoid herbal and other botanical supplements in the form of extracts, for the full synergy of the plant has a built-in safety factor compared to possible side effects of isolated plant components.

Do's

Think "synergy" and "whole food complexes" of vitamins; and "plant-derived" minerals rather than elemental minerals.

Select a foundational multi-nutrient supplement that includes a full spectrum of vitamins, chelated or plant-derived minerals, bioflavonoids, enzymes, natural food concentrates, antioxidants, whole herbs, essential fatty acids, fiber and green foods all in one formula. This will keep the amount of pills you take to a minimum and will also be easier if you need to consider your budget.

Buy a supplement that is made in an FDA compliant facility. These facilities adhere to strict quality controls from the raw material stage to the finished product.

Do buy from a responsible manufacturer with high manufacturing ethics. Research the company's mission, goals and other "About" information on their web site. Call their toll free number and ask all the questions you need to in order to decide whether you wish to buy from them. The more knowledgeable the representatives are, and the more information they disclose to you, the more transparent and trustworthy the company is.

Do remember that on a product label, the "Other Ingredients" are listed in descending order with the predominant amounts listed first down to the ingredient that is the least amount. The less ingredients listed in this area of the label, the least likely one may consume potentially allergenic, synthetic or non-nutrient substances.

Do remember it will usually take a 24-48 hour period to feel the immediate effects of a good multi-nutrient supplement, and a 30-90 day period to improve cell functioning and therefore noticeably improve your overall health.

Other than the Food and Drug Administration's (FDA) requirement that all suppliers provide the manufacturer with a Certificate of Analysis, test facilities at the manufacturer's location must test every incoming ingredient for purity and potency and reject those shipments that do not meet the high standards of Good Manufacturing Practices. Check the label for the Good Manufacturing Practices or GMP stamp. The manufacturer should be a Registered GMP facility by Nutrition Science International (NSF), the world leading authority on standards development and public safety. This distinction provides proof that the product contains what it says it does and in the potencies claimed on the label.

Choosing Your Nutritional Supplements With Confidence

You are now well informed and are ready to confidently peruse labels of virtually any nutritional supplement based on this handbook. You never again need to be persuaded about choosing less than optimal or perhaps redundant or inadequate, nonabsorbable supplements. Since you will be able to reject rather quickly many supplements and narrow your selection to the best possible choice that suits your nutritional needs, you will no longer waste time and money on incomplete or potentially toxic supplements.

You can now avoid the many synthetic vitamins and nonabsorbable minerals on the market, truly addressing your nutrient intake and experiencing quality supplementation with greater health results. Also, your superior supplement choices help ensure against nutrient deficiencies that can lead to disease, while supporting nontoxic food production methods that are sustainable and protect the environment, and ensures fair trade and ethical business practices.

Choosing nutritional supplements knowledgeably contributes to an ever expanding true health movement that works toward ensuring your health freedom and the right to know what is in your food and nutritional supplements. Your health is as good as the environment you help nurture through your wise and informed choices.

Best wishes for your true health and elevated life!

Mary Esther Miranda Gilbert

Reference:

Bano, R. "Phytosterols in Human Nutrition." *International Journal of Scientific Research and Reviews.* no. 2 (2013): 1-10. http://www.ijsrr.org/pdf/191.pdf.

Bateman, B. (2004). The effects of a double blind, placebo controlled, artificial food colourings and benzoate preservative challenge on hyperactivity in a general population sample of preschool children. *Archives of Disease in Childhood, 89*(6), doi: 10.1136/adc.2003.031435

Bischof, M. "Biophotons The Lights in Our Cells." Last modified March 2005. http://www.bibliotecapleyades.net/ciencia/ciencia_fuerz asuniverso06.htm.

Bruno, G. (2005). Bee pollen, propolis & royal jelly. *Smart Supplementation, Huntington College of Health Sciences*, Retrieved from http://www.hchs.edu/literature/Bee_ Pollen-Propolis-and-Royal_Jelly.pdf

Cancer. *Pesticide Action Network, North America*, Retrieved from http://www.panna.org/your-health/cancer

Center for Science in the Public Interest. (2013). *Chemical cuisine, learn about food additives.* Retrieved from https://www.cspinet.org/reports/chemcuisine.htm

Clement, B. (2006, December 31). *Nutri-con: the truth*

about vitamins & supplements, the vitamin myth exposed . Retrieved from http://www.organicconsumers.org/articles/article_3697.cfm

Cooke, M. Journal of the International Society of Sports Nutrition, "Effects of acute and 14-day coenzyme Q10 supplementation on exercise performance in both trained and untrained individuals." Last modified March 4, 2008. http://www.jissn.com/content/5/1/8.

Davis, J. NCHerb.Org, NC State University, "Culinary and Aromatic Herbs." Last modified April 3, 2013. http://www.ces.ncsu.edu/fletcher/programs/herbs/crops/culinary/.

Dever, J. (2013). What the science says about magnesium stearate. *Dynamic chiropractic, 31*(10), 1-4. Retrieved from http://www.progressivelabs.com/docs/DynamicChiropractic.com-What-the-Science-Says-About-Magnesium-Stearate-1372360595.pdf

Environmental Working Group. (2013). *Food additives.* Retrieved from http://www.ewg.org/search/site/food additive

European Food Safety Authority, "EFSA Panel on Dietetic Products, Nutrition and Allergies (NDA)." Last modified October 19, 2010. http://www.efsa.europa.eu/en/efsajournal/pub/1793.htm.

Fleger, K. Stanford University, Last modified 2013. http://webcache.googleusercontent.com/search?q=cac

he:http://www.ksl.stanford.edu/people/kpfleger/multivita mins/nutrients_info.txt&strip=1.

Food Chem Toxicol. 2008 Oct;46(10):3227-39. doi: 10.1016/j.fct.2008.07.024. Epub 2008 Aug 6.

George Mateljan Foundation, , "Flavonoids." Last modified October 2013. http://www.whfoods.com/genpage.php?tname=nutrient &dbid=119.

Gilbert, M. (2013, December). *How food additives affect the body.*

Godman, H. Harvard Health Publications, "LLycopene-Rich Tomatoes Linked to Lower Stroke Risk." Last modified October 10, 2012. http://www.health.harvard.edu/blog/lycopene-rich-tomatoes-linked-to-lower-stroke-risk-201210105400.

Gueye, V. (2011, January 6). The safety of natural medicine vs. conventional medicine. *Los Angeles Sentinel.* Retrieved from http://www.lasentinel.net/index.php?option=com_conte nt&view=article&id=3084:the-safety-of-natural-medicine-vs-conventional-medicine&catid=67&Itemid=157

Hance, J. (2012, March 29). Smoking gun for bee collapse? popular pesticides.

Mongabay.com, Retrieved from http://news.mongabay.com/2012/0329-hance_beecollapse_pesticides.html

Helmenstine, A. "Chemical Composition of the Human

Body." Last modified 2013.
http://chemistry.about.com/od/chemicalcomposition/a/C
hemical-Composition-Of-The-Human-Body.htm.

Higdon, Jane. Linus Pauling Institute, "Carotenoids."
Last modified June 2009.
http://lpi.oregonstate.edu/infocenter/phytochemicals/car
otenoids/.

Higdon, J. Linus Pauling Institute, "Isothiocyanates."
Last modified September 2005.
http://lpi.oregonstate.edu/infocenter/phytochemicals/iso
thio/.

Hiroyuki, M. (2012). Effect of royal jelly ingestion for six
months on healthy volunteers. *Nutrition*

Journal, 11(77), 1-7. doi: doi:10.1186/1475-2891-11-77

Hofmekler, O. (2009, July 21). *Vitamin poisoning: Are
we destroying our health with hi-potency synthetic
vitamins?*. Retrieved from
http://www.organicconsumers.org/articles/article_1861
9.cfm

Johnston, C. (2013). *Vinegar improves insulin
sensitivity to a high-carbohydrate meal in subjects with
insulin resistance or type 2 diabetes*. Retrieved from
http://care.diabetesjournals.org/content/27/1/281.full

Kobylewski, S. (2010). *Food dyes, a rainbow of risk*.
Washington, DC: Center for Science in the Public
Interest. Retrieved from http://cspinet.org/new/pdf/food-
dyes-rainbow-of-risks.pdf

Kovacs, B. (2013). *What are the different types of*

probiotics?. Retrieved from
http://www.onhealth.com/probiotics/page3.htm

Lampe, J. (2003). Spicing up a vegetarian diet:
chemopreventive effects of phytochemicals. *The American Journal of Clinical Nutrition*, *78*(3), 5798-5835. Retrieved from
http://ajcn.nutrition.org/content/78/3/579S.full

Levy, A. Citizens for Health, "Who's Afraid of Supplements; "Do You Believe in Paul Offit?"." Last modified 2013. http://www.citizens.org/save-our-supplements-do-you-believe-in-paul-offit/.

Linus Pauling Institute, "Carotenoids." Last modified 2013.
http://lpi.oregonstate.edu/infocenter/phytochemicals/carotenoids/.

Linus Pauling Institute, "Chlorophyll and Chlorophyllin."
Last modified June 2009.
http://lpi.oregonstate.edu/infocenter/phytochemicals/chlorophylls/.

Linus Pauling Institute. (2013). *Flavonoids*. Retrieved from
http://lpi.oregonstate.edu/infocenter/phytochemicals/flavonoids/

Linus Pauling Institute, Oregon State University, "Garlic and Organosulfur Compounds." Last modified 2013.
http://lpi.oregonstate.edu/infocenter/phytochemicals/garlic/index.html.

Linus Pauling Institute, "Vitamin C." Last modified 2013.

http://lpi.oregonstate.edu/infocenter/vitamins/vitaminC/i
ndex.html.

Medicinal Plants. (2011). *Herb-drug interactions:
natural coumarins*. Retrieved from
http://medicinalplants.us/herb-drug-interactions-natural-
coumarins

Medline Plus, U.S. National Library of Medicine,
National Institutes of Health, "Acetaminophen." Last
modified October 30, 2013.
http://www.nlm.nih.gov/medlineplus/druginfo/meds/a68
1004.html.

Medline Plus, U.S. National Library of Medicine,
National Institutes of Health, "Aspirin." Last modified
October 30, 2013.
http://www.nlm.nih.gov/medlineplus/druginfo/meds/a68
2878.html

Mohankumar, A. "Production and Characterization of
Serratiopeptidase Enzyme from Serratia Marcescens."
International Journal of Biology. no. 3 (2011): 1-13.
www.ccsenet.org/journal/index.php/ijb/article/download
/11170/7883.doi:10.5539/ijb.v3n3p39

National Cancer Institute, National Institutes of Health,
"Questions and Answers About Coenzyme Q10." Last
modified 2 19, 2013.
http://www.cancer.gov/cancertopics/pdq/cam/coenzym
eQ10/patient/page2.

National Center for Complementary and Alternative
Medicine, (2008). *Two studies explore the potential
health benefits of probiotics*. Retrieved from website:
http://nccam.nih.gov/research/results/spotlight/110508.

htm

National Institute of Diabetes and Digestive and Kidney Diseases, National Diabetes Information Clearinghouse. (2013). *Insulin resistance and prediabetes, what happens with insulin resistance?*. Retrieved from website: http://diabetes.niddk.nih.gov/dm/pubs/insulinresistance/

NOSG, Naturally Occurring Standards Group. (n.d.). Retrieved from http://www.nosg.org/index.html

Office of Dietary Supplements, National Institutes of Health, "Dietary Supplement Fact Sheet Selenium." Last modified July 2, 2013. http://ods.od.nih.gov/factsheets/VitaminC-QuickFacts/.

Office of Dietary Supplements, National Institutes of Health, "Dietary Supplement Fact Sheet Vitamin C." http://ods.od.nih.gov/factsheets/VitaminC-QuickFacts/.

Office of Dietary Supplements, National Institutes of Health, "Dietary Supplement Fact Sheet Vitamin E." Last modified June 5, 2013. http://ods.od.nih.gov/factsheets/VitaminE-HealthProfessional/.

Office of Dietary Supplements, National Insitutes of Health, "Zinc Dietary Supplement Fact Sheet." http://ods.od.nih.gov/factsheets/Zinc-HealthProfessional/.

O'Hara, A. (2006). The gut flora as a forgotten organ. *EMBO Reports, 7*, 688-693. doi: doi:10.1038/sj.embor.7400731

Panayota, M. (2010). *Vinegar decreases postprandial hyperglycemia in patients with type 1 diabetes.* Retrieved from http://care.diabetesjournals.org/content/33/2/e27.full

Pesticide Action Network, North America. (2010). *12 pesticide residues found by the usda pesticide data program.* Retrieved from http://www.whatsonmyfood.org/food.jsp?food=HY

Pettis, J. (2013). Crop pollination exposes honey bees to pesticides which alters their susceptibility to the gut pathogen nosema ceranae . *PLOS One*, doi: •DOI: 10.1371/journal.pone.0070182

Phytochemicals. (n.d.). *List of phytochemicals.* Retrieved from http://www.phytochemicals.info/phytochemicals.php

Phytochemicals, "Proanthocyanidins." http://www.phytochemicals.info/phytochemicals/proant hocyanidins.php.

Phytochemicals, "Resveratrol." http://www.phytochemicals.info/phytochemicals/resvera trol.php.

Rowett Research Institute, "Fact Sheet, Body Composition." http://www.rowett.ac.uk/edu_web/sec_pup/body_comp. pdf.

Schmid, R. (2002). *More background information on good and bad ingredients found in vitamins and supplements. Additives.* Retrieved from http://www.organicconsumers.org/articles/article_4322.

cfm

Shan, B. (2005). Antioxidant capacity of 26 spice extracts and characterization of their phenolic constituents. *Journal of Agricultural Food Chemistry, 53*(20), 7749-7759. doi: DOI: 10.1021/jf051513y

Singh, V. (2013). Role of probiotics in health and disease: a review. *The Journal of the Pakistan Medical Association, 63*(2), 253-7. Retrieved from http://www.ncbi.nlm.nih.gov/pubmed/23894906

Stanford University, "The Consumer Guide to Multi-Vitamins." Last modified 2000. http://www.ksl.stanford.edu/people/kpfleger/multivitamins/cached/www.mothernature.com_cg_multi_vitamins.asp.html.

Tacouri, D. (2013). In vitro bioactivity and phytochemical screening of selected spices used. *Asian Pacific Journal of Tropical Disease, 3*(4), 253-261. doi: 10.1016/S2222-1808(13)60066-3

Tapparo, A. (2012). Assessment of the environmental exposure of honeybees to particulate matter containing neonicotinoid insecticides coming from corn coated seeds. *Environmental Science & Technology, 46*(5), 2592-9. doi: 10.1021/es2035152

UCLA, History Special Collections, Louise M. Daring Biomedical Library. (2002). *Chemicals in spices.* Retrieved from http://unitproj.library.ucla.edu/biomed/spice/index.cfm?spicefilename=activeProperties.txt&itemsuppress=yes&displayswitch=0

UCLA History & Special Collections, Louise M. Darling Biomedical Library. (2002). *Medical use of spices*. Retrieved from http://unitproj.library.ucla.edu/biomed/spice/index.cfm?spicefilename=medspice.txt&itemsuppress=yes&displayswitch=0

University of Maryland Medical Center. (2013, May 7). *Bromelain*. Retrieved from http://umm.edu/health/medical/altmed/supplement/bromelain

University of Maryland Medical Center, "CoEnzyme Q10." Last modified 2011. http://umm.edu/health/medical/altmed/supplement/coenzyme-q10.

U.S. Food and Drug Administration, The U.S. Department of Health and Human Services, "Guidance for Industry: Current Good Manufacturing Practice in Manufacturing, Packaging, Labeling, or Holding Operations for Dietary Supplements; Small Entity Compliance Guide." Last modified December 2010. http://www.fda.gov/Food/GuidanceRegulation/GuidanceDocumentsRegulatoryInformation/DietarySupplements/ucm238182.htm.

Williams, C. (n.d.). *Hungry kids: fill them up with healthy high-fiber foods*. Retrieved from http://www.nationalfibercouncil.org/pdfs/Hungry_Kids.pdf

Woyengo, T. "Anticancer effects of phytosterols." *European Journal of Clinical Nutrition*. no. 7 (2009): 813-20. http://www.ncbi.nlm.nih.gov/pubmed/19491917.

Wu, G. "Glutathione metabolism and its implications for health." *The Journal of Nutrition.* no. 3 (2004): 389-92. http://www.ncbi.nlm.nih.gov/pubmed/14988435.

Zelman, K. (n.d.). *The benefits of fiber: for your heart, weight and energy.* Retrieved from http://www.webmd.com/diet/fiber-health-benefits-11/insoluble-soluble-fiber

Mary Esther Miranda Gilbert

Appendix
Further Information and Resources

Websites:

www.HolisticChoices.com

www.holisticchoices.com/The-True-Health-Journal.html

Other Books by the Author:
True Health Mastery: Transform Your Health; Change the World
The Ten Tenets of True Health
The Cross Country Athlete

Other Works by the Author:
Publishing Editor, The True Health Journal
Founder, CEO, The True Health Academy

True Health Mastery Series of Online Courses:

- Holistic Nutrition 101 - Nutritional Synergy™© Deliciously Ultimate Health and Lifelong Vibrancy
- Family Obesity - Preventing Family Crisis
- Sports Nutrition For Athletes - Consistent Performance, Avoiding Fatigue, Burnout, Injuries, Faster Healing and More Complete Recovery
- Weight Management Mastery - The Real Reasons For The Weight Loss Struggle
- For Bridal Couples: Healthy Beginnings; Your Future Legacy

Mary Esther Miranda Gilbert

ABOUT THE AUTHOR

With over 35 years experience as a nutrition science physiology and alternative medicine research writer, the author has educated her clients and audiences about the essential connection between understanding and applying complete and correct nutrition, and mastering one's health--for life.

The author is an honors graduate of the Clayton College of Natural Health, having earned a Bachelor and Master of Science Degree in Holistic Nutrition. She is also a summa cum laude honors graduate of Kaplan University with a Bachelors degree in Nutrition Science. She is a member of the International Golden Key Honor Society, and the Alpha Beta Kappa Honor Society and Alumni of Kaplan University. She has been a long-standing member of the American Holistic Health Association and the American Association of Nutritional Consultants.

She is currently active in educating the public with the knowledge needed for profound, positive change in the many destructive aspects of our modern world that affects all living things within the Earth's critical ecology.